SELF-ASSESSMENT PICTURE TESTS IN DENTISTRY

PEDIATRIC DENTISTRY

Edited by
L. SHAW
BDS, PhD, LDS, FDS, RCS (Eng)
The University of Birmingham Dental School,
Birmingham, England

M WOLFE

Copyright © 1994 Mosby–Year Book Europe Ltd
Published in 1994 by Wolfe Publishing.
Reprinted 1995 by Mosby–Wolfe, an imprint of Times Mirror International Publisherz Ltd

Printed in Spain by Grafos, S.A. ARTE SOBRE PAPEL

ISBN 0 7234 1929 9

For full details of all Mosby titles please write to Times Mirror International Publishing Lt
Lynton House, 7–12 Tavistock Square, London WC1H 9LB, England.

A CIP catalogue record for this book is available from the British Library.

Library of Congress Cataloging-in-Publication Data
Linda Shaw
     Self-assessment picture tests in dentistry: pedodontics / Linda Shaw.
          p. cm.
       ISBN 0-7234-1929-9
       1. Pedodontics—Examinations, questions, etc. 2. Pedodontics—
—Atlases. I. Title.
       [DNLM: 1. Pediatric Dentistry—examination questions,
     2. Pediatric Dentistry—atlases. WU 18 S535s 1993]
     RK55, C5S52 1993
     617.6'45'0076—dc20
     DNLM/DLC
     for Library of Congress   93-8372
                                                                  CIP

PREFACE

Any man who reads too much and uses his brain too little falls into lazy habits of thinking.

Albert Einstein

I hope that this is a book to be opened with anticipation and closed with profit. It consists of a wide range of questions and answers on common and uncommon paediatric dental problems. These are arranged in random order, although some have a deliberately longitudinal theme to check whether information has been assimilated! It is intended that they cover a range of subjects that will test the undergraduate, extend the practitioner and stimulate the postgraduate. It should encourage the use of the brain in logical deduction and activate thought whilst reading—making Einsteins of all of us!

ACKNOWLEDGEMENTS

Sincere thanks are due to April Gallett for her efficient preparation of the manuscript; the photographic departments of all the contributors' hospitals are gratefully acknowledged. Permission was kindly given by the editors of the *British Dental Journal* and *Dental Update* for reproduction of figures.

LIST OF CONTRIBUTORS

R. Bedi, BDS, MSc, FDSRCS Ed
The University of Birmingham Dental School, Birmingham, England.
P.J.M. Crawford, BDS, MScD, FDSRCS Ed
The University of Bristol, England.
J.R. Goodman, BDS, FDSRCS Eng
Eastman Dental Hospital, Institute of Dental Surgery, The University of London, England.
M.C. Grundy, LDS, DDS, FDSRCS Eng
The University of Birmingham Dental School, Birmingham, England.
F.J. Hill, BDS, MDS, FDSRCPS Glasg, DOrth RCS
Turner Dental School, The University of Manchester, England.
R.D. Holt, BChD, MSc, PhD
Institute of Dental Surgery, The University of London, England.
I.C. Mackie, BDS, MSc, PhD, DDPHRCS, FDSRCPS Glasg.
Turner Dental School, The University of Manchester, England.
J.H. Nunn, BDS, DDPHRCS, PhD, FDSRCS Edin
The Dental School, The University of Newcastle upon Tyne, Newcastle upon Tyne, England.
G.J. Roberts, BDS, PhD, MDS, FDSRCS Eng
United Medical and Dental Schools, Guy's Hospital Dental School, The University of London, England.
W.P. Rock, BDS, DDS, LDS, DOrth RCS, FDSRCS Eng.
The University of Birmingham Dental School, Birmingham, England.
A.J. Rugg-Gunn, RD, DSc, BDS, PhD, FDSRCS Ed
The Dental School, The University of Newcastle upon Tyne, Newcastle upon Tyne, England.
L. Shaw, BDS, PhD, LDS, FDSRCS Eng.
The University of Birmingham Dental School, Birmingham, England.
R.R. Welbury, MBBS, BDS, PhD, FDSRCS Eng.
The Dental School, The University of Newcastle upon Tyne, Newcastle upon Tyne, England.

QUESTIONS

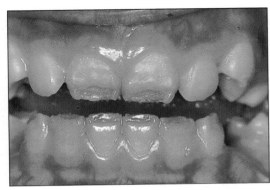

Figure 1

1 The permanent incisor teeth (*Figure 1*) of this 10-year-old girl are defective.
(a) What is the possible cause?
(b) Why are the upper lateral incisors not affected?
(c) Which other teeth may be affected?
(d) How would you treat these teeth?

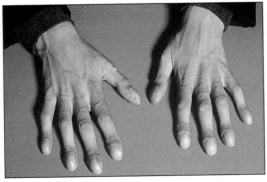

Figure 2

2 (a) What clinical sign does *Figure 2* show?
(b) What conditions is it associated with?

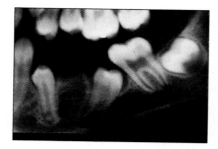

3 (a) Comment on the alignment of the mandibular teeth shown in this radiograph (*Figure 3*).
(b) How might this unsatisfactory alignment have been avoided by different management at an earlier stage?

Figure 3

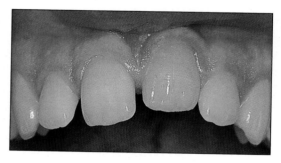

Figure 4

4 The upper left permanent central incisor in this patient is shorter than the contralateral tooth (*Figure 4*).
(a) What is the probable cause?
(b) What investigations are necessary, and what results would you expect?
(c) What treatment would you carry out?

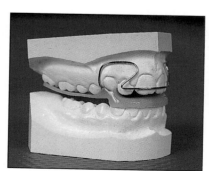

5 (a) What is the name of this appliance (*Figure 5*)?
(b) Upon what factors is case selection normally based?
(c) What is the most undesirable occlusal change that tends to result from treatment with these appliances? How is it prevented?

Figure 5

6 (a) What is the most likely nature of the lesion shown in this radiograph (*Figure 6*)?
(b) Could this problem have been avoided?
(c) Outline the essentials of management which are now necessary to ensure eruption of the permanent upper right central incisor.

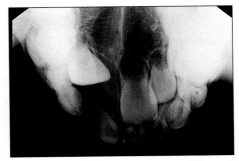

Figure 6

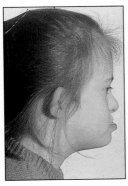

Figure 7

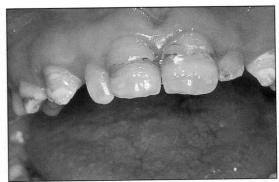

Figure 8

7 (a) Which syndrome does this child suffer from (*Figure 7*)?
(b) What is the epidemiology of the condition?
(c) Identify the extra-oral and intra-oral (*Figure 8*) features of the syndrome in this child.
(d) What other features are associated with this syndrome?

8 (a) What are the chief clinical characteristics of 'rampant' or 'nursing bottle' caries?
(b) Which groups of children are thought to be at particular risk of developing this form of caries?

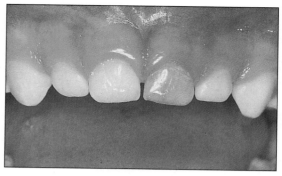

Figure 9

9 This 4-year-old child presented with discoloration of the upper left incisor (*Figure 9*) and has a history of a fall a year ago.
(a) Discuss the prevalence of the injury you see and your management of the child.
(b) What are the sequelae of this type of injury to the permanent dentition?

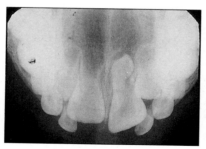

Figure 10

10 This occlusal radiograph (*Figure 10*) was taken as part of a routine investigation of a child's developing dentition.
(a) Comment fully on the abnormality shown by the radiograph.
(b) How would you initially manage this problem in a healthy and co-operative child with no associated symptoms?
(c) Is any further treatment likely to be necessary later?

11 (a) Which of the following trace elements are considered to affect dental caries experience?

Fluorine, Iron, Molybdenum, Strontium, Iodine, Selenium

(b) Which are thought to inhibit caries, and which promote caries?
(c) On what kind of evidence are those views based, and how extensive is the evidence?

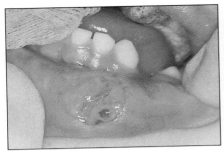

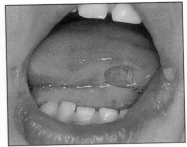

Figure 11

Figure 12

12 This 2-year-old cerebral palsied child has caused extensive damage to her oral soft tissues by biting (*Figures 11* and *12*). What is the likely cause, and how would you manage this condition?

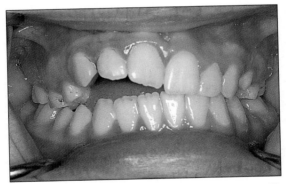

Figure 13

13 (a) What is this occlusal abnormality (*Figure 13*) and what is the most likely cause?
(b) What other occlusal anomaly is often associated with this condition, and how is it produced?
(c) How should the condition be managed?

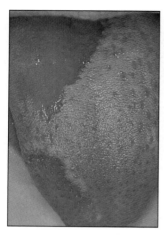

14 The parent of this child is worried about the lesion on his tongue (*Figure 14*).
(a) What is the lesion?
(b) What is the aetiology?
(c) What is the prognosis?

Figure 14

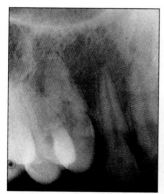

Figure 15

15 This teenager had the right upper canine (3|) transplanted two years ago.
(a) Describe the appearance shown in *Figures 15* and *16*.
(b) How would you manage this patient?

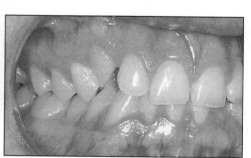

Figure 16

16 The Department of Health (London) has set out guidelines for nutrient intakes in the United Kingdom.
(a) In what years were there major reports on: (i) cardiovascular disease; (ii) dietary sugars; (iii) dietary reference values?
(b) What were the main recommendations of these reports?

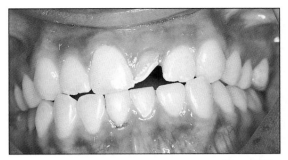

Figure 17

17 The left upper central incisor of this patient (*Figure 17*) was fractured four years previously and has been satisfactorily root filled. The patient is now 15 years old and requests a restoration to improve his appearance.
(a) Comment on the difficulties of providing a crown for this tooth.
(b) What treatment is required before a successful crown can be provided?
(c) Could this difficult problem have been avoided by different earlier management?

Figure 18

18 *Figure 18* illustrates the results of a famous study on the relationship between the level of fluoride in drinking water and dental caries experience.
(a) Who was the author of this study, where was it carried out, and in what decade?
(b) What is the main conclusion from this figure and how has it influenced water fluoridation policy?

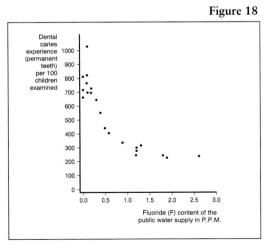

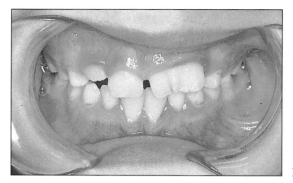

Figure 19

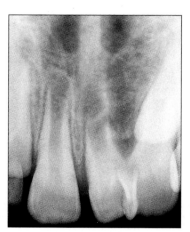

19 (a) What is the condition illustrated in these clinical and radiograph pictures (*Figures 19* and *20*)?
(b) What are the problems which may arise as a result of this condition?
(c) What is the treatment of choice?

Figure 20

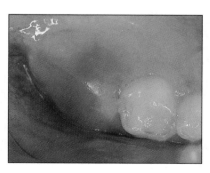

20 (a) What is the likely nature of this swelling in the first permanent molar region (*Figure 21*)?
(b) What is the cause?
(c) What treatment is necessary?

Figure 21

21 (a) How may caries be diagnosed in the young child?
(b) What are the disadvantages of these methods?

22 The central incisor tooth in this 9 year old suffered a crown fracture, producing a large exposure of the pulp (*Figure 22*). Presentation was delayed for 24 hours.
(a) What treatment would you carry out, assuming that the patient is both healthy and co-operative?
(b) What is the prognosis for success?

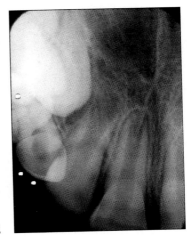

Figure 22

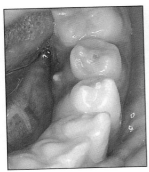

Figure 23

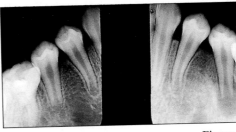

Figure 24

23 A 12-year-old Japanese girl presented with the condition shown in *Figure 23*, complaining that the lower left second premolar was painful and tender to pressure. The radiographic appearance of this tooth and of the lower premolars is shown in *Figure 24*.
(a) What is the diagnosis?
(b) Is the patient's nationality of any significance?
(c) Outline how you would manage this problem, assuming a healthy and co-operative patient with a good occlusion.

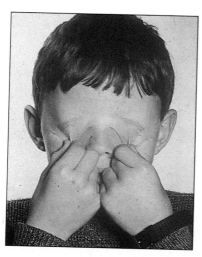

24 (a) From which syndrome does this boy suffer (*Figure 25*)?
(b) What are the main clinical features?
(c) What major complication of this syndrome is important when considering dental treatment?

Figure 25

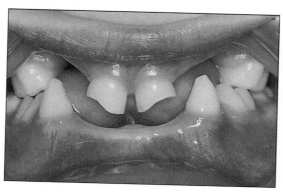

Figure 26

25 This 6-year-old boy (*Figure 26*) was referred for advice on treatment for his hypodontia. The following teeth were absent:

$$\frac{5432 \mid 2345}{54\ 21\mid 12\ 45}$$

(a) What is the prevalence of this condition and which teeth are most frequently missing?
(b) What other oral and general conditions are sometimes associated with hypodontia?
(c) What is the treatment rationale in these cases?

26 (a) What are the common sequelae of rampant caries?
(b) What are the major principles of treatment of this form of caries?

27 *Figure 27* shows the periapical radiograph of the tooth shown in *Figure 22*, two years post-treatment.
(a) Which radiographic signs indicate that the treatment has been successful?
(b) The tooth does not respond to pulpal vitality testing. Would this influence your management?

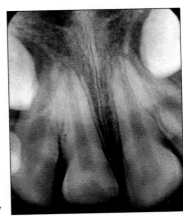

Figure 27

28 This 6-month-old baby (*Figure 28*) knocked his lower primary incisors with a spoon.
(a) What treatment would you carry out?
(b) Give your reasons.

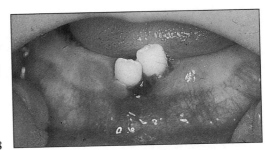

Figure 28

29 (a) What is the soft tissue lesion shown here (*Figure 29*)?
(b) Classify and describe the lesion histologically.
(c) How should it be treated?

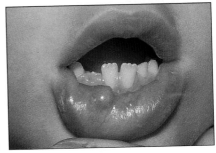

Figure 29

Figure 30

Mean decay incidence for children of different ages in England in 1983					
	Permanent decay experience				
Age	D	M	F	DMF	% caries free
8	0.3	0.0	0.4	0.7	65
12	0.6	0.3	2.0	2.9	21
15	0.9	0.5	4.2	5.6	8

30 (a) What is the accepted method of measuring the prevalence of dental caries in permanent teeth that has been used in *Figure 30*?
(b) What are the disadvantages of this method?

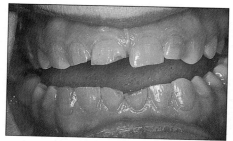

31 (a) What condition is affecting the teeth of this 16-year-old boy (*Figure 31*)?
(b) How would you confirm your diagnosis?
(c) What treatment would you advise for him?
(d) What is the prognosis?

Figure 31

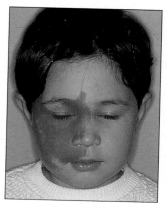

32 (a) What is the condition shown in *Figure 32*?
(b) It may, on rare occasions, be associated with which other condition?
(c) How does it affect dental care?

Figure 32

Figure 33

33 This patient's upper first premolar (*Figure 33*) shows an enamel defect. There are no similar defects elsewhere in the dentition.
(a) What is the likely nature and cause of this defect?
(b) How can the occurrence of such defects be minimised?
(c) How could the appearance of the premolar be improved?

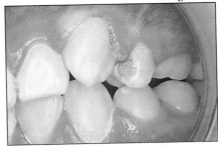

34 (a) What do you see on this radiograph (*Figure 34*)?
(b) What treatment would you carry out in order to conserve this tooth?
(c) What is the reported success rate of this treatment?

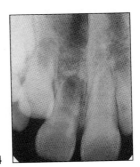

Figure 34

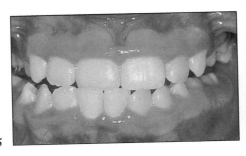

Figure 35

35 This extremely nervous 11-year-old girl (*Figures 35* and *36*) is asplenic, has a right hemiplegia and a congenital heart defect requiring antibiotic cover. She is taking penicillin prophylactically and is allergic to erythromycin. She requires extensive scaling of her teeth to remove sub-gingival calculus and occlusal restorations to her first permanent molars. How would you manage her dental care?

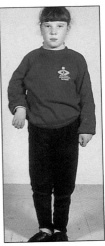

Figure 36

36 (a) What changes occurred at a national level in the UK during 1990, which had a major impact on the delivery of dental care for children?
(b) How might these changes affect dental care for children and how might this be monitored?

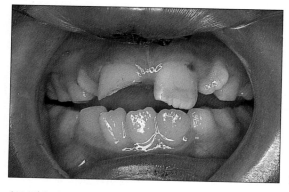

Figure 37

37 This 9-year-old boy presented one hour after an accident which resulted in the coronal fracture and small pulpal exposure shown in *Figure 37*.
(a) What treatment would you carry out on the tooth?
(b) What is the reported success rate of this treatment?

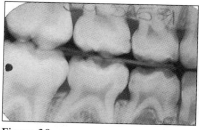

Figure 38   Figure 39

38 These bite-wing radiographs (*Figures 38* and *39*) are of a 6-year-old girl who had previously had a caries-free dentition.
(a) What investigations would you carry out?
(b) What treatment would you advise?

39 (a) What is the lesion on the mandibular gingiva of this 7-day-old infant likely to be (*Figure 40*)?
(b) What are its histological features?
(c) How should it be treated?

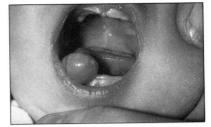

Figure 40

40 (a) What significant features does this boy exhibit (*Figure 41*)?
(b) With what condition are they associated?
(c) What is the aetiology?
(d) What oral problems might you expect to find?

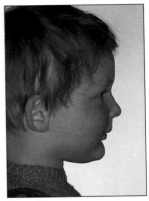

Figure 41

41 This 2-year-old child (*Figure 42*) hit her mouth against a coffee table.
(a) What is the reported incidence of trauma to primary teeth?
(b) How would you treat this child?
(c) What advice should you give the parents?
(d) What secondary injuries might be sustained by the permanent successor?

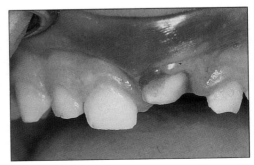

Figure 42

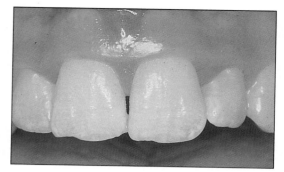

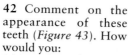

42 Comment on the appearance of these teeth (*Figure 43*). How would you:
(a) investigate the cause?
(b) classify the appearance?
(c) treat the teeth?

Figure 43

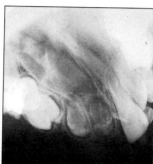

43 This radiograph (*Figure 44*) shows an indistinct area in the upper left anterior region.
(a) What is the diagnosis of this condition?
(b) How may it be managed?

Figure 44

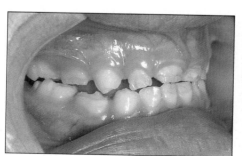

44 (a) What condition is affecting the primary teeth in this patient (*Figure 45*)?
(b) How might it have been caused?
(c) What features help in the differential diagnosis?

Figure 45

45 (a) What general condition is illustrated by this patient's radiograph (*Figure 46*)?
(b) How should the dental problems be managed?

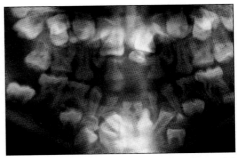

Figure 46

46 The right upper central incisor of this 14-year-old boy was replanted 4 years ago (*Figure 47*).
(a) What is the condition called?
(b) How has the problem arisen?
(c) What treatment would be appropriate to improve the appearance of the anterior teeth?
(d) How would you try to avoid this happening in replanted teeth?

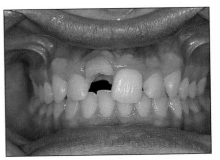

Figure 47

47 (a) Which of the ingredients in this food label (*Figure 48*) are non-sugar sweeteners?
(b) Are these bulk or intense sweeteners?
(c) List six bulk and four intense sweeteners allowed for use in foods in the UK in 1992.

INGREDIENTS

Isomalt, Full Cream Milk Powder, Cocoa Butter Emulsifier (Lecithin), Flavourings, Artificial Sweetener (Aspartame), Colour (Curcumin).

Contains Phenylalanine

Figure 48

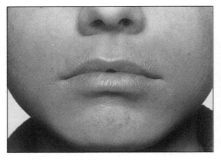

48 A skin rash appeared on the face of this young boy (*Figure 49*) a few days after a fixed bonded orthodontic appliance had been fitted.
(a) What is the likely diagnosis?
(b) What mechanism is involved?
(c) What action should be taken?

Figure 49

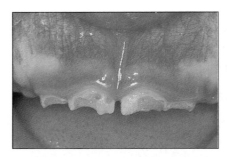

49 This 3-year-old child (*Figure 50*) has been raised on a largely sugar-free diet.
(a) What could have given rise to this appearance?
(b) How should it be managed?

Figure 50

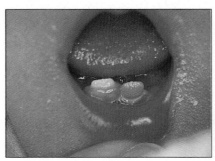

Figure 51

50 This newborn baby (*Figure 51*) was found to have teeth present.
(a) What is the difference between a natal and neonatal tooth?
(b) How common are natal teeth?

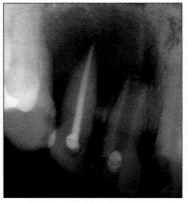

Figure 52

51 Approximately how old is this patient (*Figure 52*)?

52 (a) What oral abnormalities can be seen in this patient (*Figure 53*)?
(b) How would you manage the soft tissue problems?

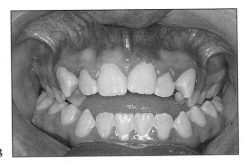

Figure 53

53 (a) Describe the lesion you see on the left-hand side of the face, neck and intra-oral area of this 5-year-old girl (*Figures 54* and *55*).
(b) What are the aims of dental care?
(c) What are some of the problems associated with the defect?

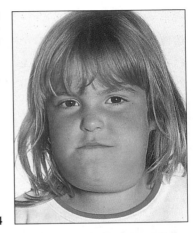

Figure 54

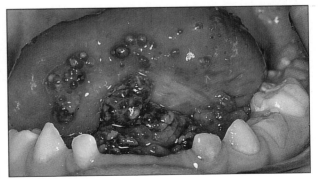

Figure 55

54 What aetiological factors have been identified as important in rampant caries?

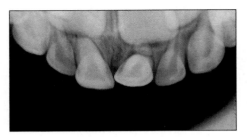

Figure 56

55 This 4-year-old child fell 3 hours previous to presentation.
(a) Describe what you see on the radiograph (*Figure 56*).
(b) What treatment options would you consider?

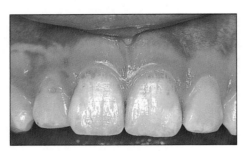

Figure 57

56 (a) What abnormality is shown in the cervical areas of these incisors (*Figure 57*)?
(b) What is its cause?
(c) What treatment is needed?

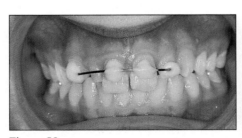

Figure 58   Figure 59

57 (a) What materials could be used to produce this splint (*Figures 58* and *59*)?
(b) What are the recommended splinting periods for a replanted tooth, subluxed tooth, displaced tooth which has been repositioned, and a tooth with a root fracture?

58 (a) How may caries be predicted in the young child?
(b) How accurate are the available methods of prediction for a young child patient?

59 This girl and her mother have regular recurrent gingivitis, together with skin infections (*Figure 60*).
(a) What is the condition?
(b) Why does it occur?

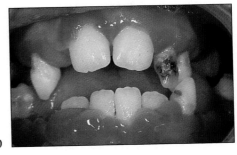

Figure 60

60 This is an extreme case, affecting a lower canine tooth, of a condition that frequently affects upper permanent incisor teeth (*Figure 61*).
(a) What is the condition?
(b) What are the signs of its presence in incisors and to what problems can it give rise?

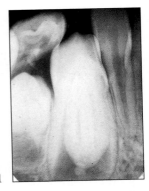

Figure 61

61 This condition affected the primary and permanent dentitions equally (*Figure 62*).
(a) What is this condition called?
(b) What dental radiographic findings would you expect to see?

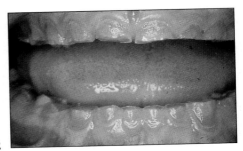

Figure 62

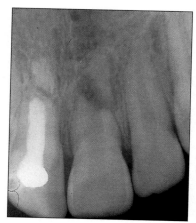

62 (a) Describe what you see on this radiograph (*Figure 63*).
(b) How would you treat this patient?

Figure 63

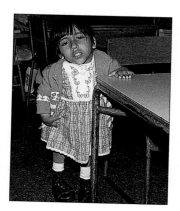

63 This 6-year-old girl is very small for her age (*Figure 64*).
(a) What condition does she suffer from?
(b) What is its aetiology and prevalence?
(c) What are the typical facial and oral findings?

Figure 64

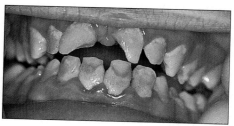

64 This 13-year-old boy has severe learning difficulties and epilepsy.
(a) What dental problems are apparent (*Figure 65*)?
(b) How would you manage his dental care?

Figure 65

65 You are asked to examine a 2-day-old baby who has a slightly loose natal tooth (*Figure 66*). The mother is concerned that the tooth may be swallowed or inhaled if left. How would you manage this case?

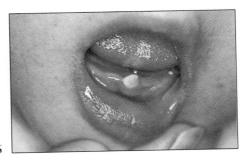

Figure 66

66 This referred 13-year-old has a history of recurrent abscess associated with the right upper central incisor. The referral letter asks for an apicectomy to be carried out.
(a) What do you see on the radiograph (*Figure 67*)?
(b) Do you think that an apicectomy is indicated?
(c) What alternative treatment would be indicated?

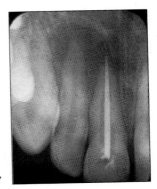

Figure 67

67 Many developed countries have reported dramatic reductions in the prevalence of dental caries in the last two decades (*Figure 68*).
(a) What global dental goals have been set by the World Health Organization for children and young adults, to be achieved by the year 2000?
(b) What are some of the reasons suggested for this decline in dental disease?

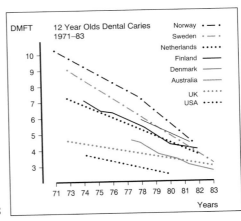

Figure 68

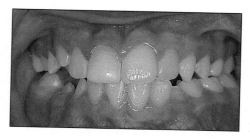

Figure 69

68 This young patient (*Figure 69*) has had a pulp-capping procedure carried out on the right upper central incisor and this has been scheduled for review in 6 months.
(a) What points would you look for in the review examination?
(b) What special tests would you carry out?

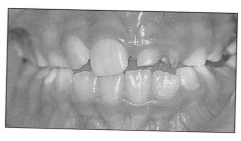

Figure 70

69 The maxillary left central and lateral incisors have failed to erupt in this 9-year-old child (*Figure 70*).
(a) What is the most likely cause of the eruption failure?
(b) What investigations would you carry out in order to establish a diagnosis?
(c) What treatment is required if the diagnosis is confirmed?

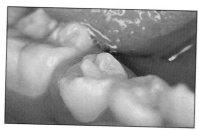

70 (a) What is the anomaly shown in *Figure 71* called?
(b) What problems can be associated with it?
(c) What teeth are affected and is there any associated gender or racial bias?

Figure 71

71 (a) What condition is indicated by the appearance of the hands of this child (*Figure 72*)?
(b) What is its mode of inheritance?
(c) What are the oral complications of this condition?
(d) What is the treatment?

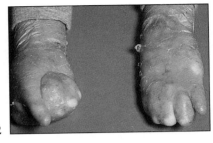

Figure 72

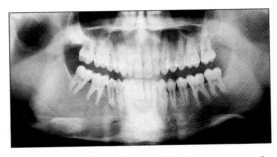

Figure 73

72 (a) What is the bony abnormality in the right mandibular ramus, angle and body of this teenager (*Figure 73*)?
(b) How would you describe the radiological texture of the affected bone?
(c) What is the treatment?

73 This 3-year-old child fell 30 minutes prior to presentation (*Figure 74*). The left upper primary central incisor could not be found at the scene of the accident.
(a) What questions would you ask the parent, bearing in mind that the tooth is unaccounted for?
(b) What special tests would you carry out?
(c) What treatment would you recommend?

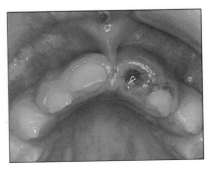

Figure 74

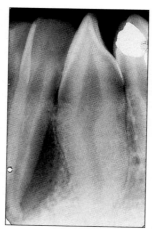

74 This patient (*Figure 75*) has had multiple non-vital teeth with no obvious dental cause, but related to his inherited metabolic disorder.
(a) What is the condition?
(b) What does the radiograph show?
(c) What is the histological appearance of the teeth?

Figure 75

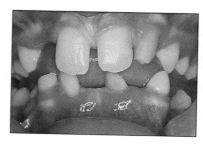

75 This patient complains about the appearance of her teeth, which she has cared for well (*Figure 76*).
(a) What is the name of this condition?
(b) What is its prevalence?
(c) What is its sex distribution?

Figure 76

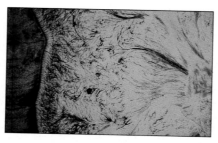

Figure 77

76 (a) What type of histologic section is this (*Figure 77*)?
(b) Describe what it shows.
(c) What is your diagnosis?

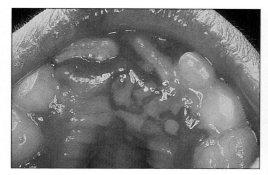
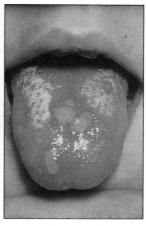

Figure 78

Figure 79

77 This 6-year-old child has a fever, is unwell and complains of a sore mouth (*Figures 78* and *79*).
(a) What is the diagnosis?
(b) Give the other clinical features likely to be associated.
(c) How is it transmitted?
(d) How would you manage this patient?

78 Glass ionomer (poly-alkenoate) cement was first developed in 1972, and has been used increasingly in paediatric practice.
(a) What reaction is its chemical constitution based on?
(b) Which properties make it useful in clinical paediatric dentistry?

79 (a) What type of radiograph is this (*Figure 80*)?
(b) What main feature does it show?
(c) What condition is this treatment associated with?
(d) What is the significance for dental treatment?

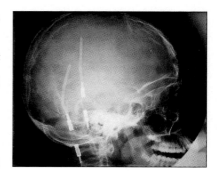

Figure 80

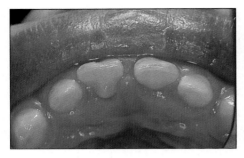

80 (a) What is this anomaly (*Figure 81*)?
(b) How common is it?
(c) Are any other anomalies associated with this condition?

Figure 81

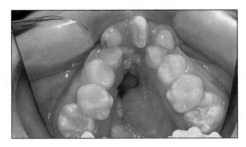

81 (a) What condition is present in this 6-year-old boy (*Figure 82*)?
(b) What is its incidence?
(c) What are the objectives of interdisciplinary care?

Figure 82

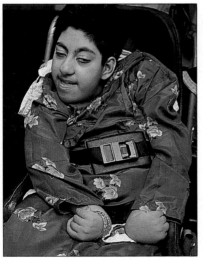

82 This 12-year-old girl has cerebral palsy (*Figure 83*).
(a) Describe this condition.
(b) How is it classified?
(c) What implications does this have for dental care?

Figure 83

83 (a) Describe this traumatic injury (*Figure 84*).
(b) How would you treat this patient?
(c) What complications would you look for during follow-up?

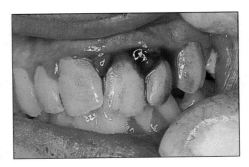

Figure 84

84 (a) What type of radiographic film(*Figure 85*) has been produced in answer to a request for a vertex occlusal?
(b) The film was requested to permit accurate positioning of an unerupted canine before the tooth was surgically exposed. What would be the diagnosis if this film was relied upon?
(c) Why is the use of the vertex occlusal view to be discouraged?

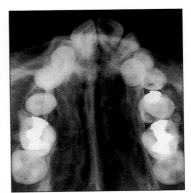

Figure 85

85 A mother is concerned that her one week old baby has an ulcer on the base of its tongue and is feeding with difficulty (*Figure 86*).
(a) What is the cause of this ulcer?
(b) How would you manage the situation?

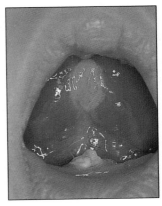

Figure 86

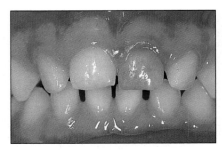

86 (a) What do you see in this photograph (*Figure 87*)?
(b) What special tests would you advise?
(c) How does your treatment depend upon the results of the special tests?

Figure 87

87 What are the main methods suitable for preventing caries in the young child patient?

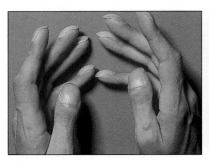 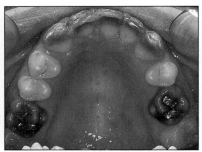

Figure 88   **Figure 89**

88 (a) What is the condition shown in this teenager (*Figures 88* and *89*)?
(b) Why do his fingers appear as they do?
(c) Comment on the dental features seen in this patient.

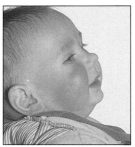

89 (a) Comment on the appearance of this baby (*Figure 90*), who is also mentally handicapped.
(b) List the possible causes of mental handicap.

Figure 90

90 (a) What is the most likely cause of this hypoplastic central incisor (*Figure 91*)?
(b) At what age was the cause operative?
(c) What treatment is indicated?

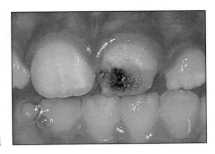

Figure 91

91 (a) What is evident on this radiograph (*Figure 92*)?
(b) What treatment would you recommend for this patient?

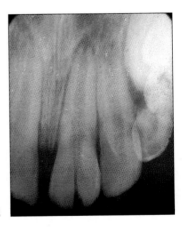

Figure 92

92 (a) Describe the condition shown in *Figure 93*.
(b) How would you manage this patient?

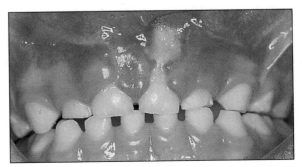

Figure 93

Figure 94   **Figure 95**

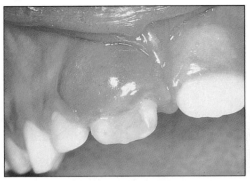 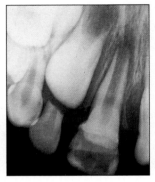

93 This patient presented with an acute infection (*Figures* 94 and 95).
(a) What is this condition?
(b) What is the probable aetiology?
(c) What does the radiograph indicate?

94 For which groups of young child patients would you recommend the following preventive measures:
(a) Fluoride drops or tablets
(b) Fluoride-containing toothpastes
(c) Fluoride varnish applications
(d) Dietary restriction of sugar intake?

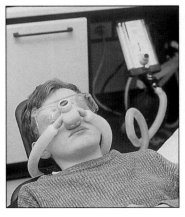

95 List the indications and contra-indications for relative analgesia (*Figure 96*).

Figure 96

96 This 12-year-old girl (*Figure* 97) has buccally displaced canine teeth in an otherwise uncrowded dentition. Describe your treatment plan, with supporting justification.

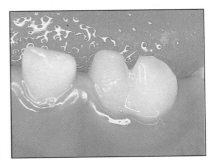

Figure 97

97 (a) What is the name of this anomaly in the mandibular canine region (*Figure* 98)?
(b) What is its prevalence?

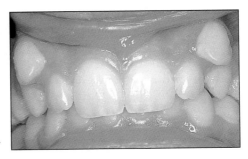

Figure 98

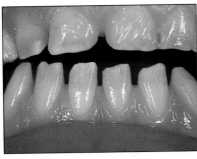

Figure 99

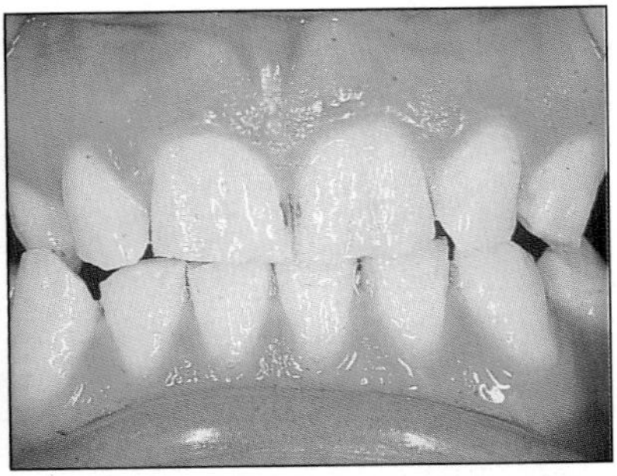

Figure 100

98 *Figures* 99 and 100 show a male and female affected by the same condition.
(a) What is the condition?
(b) Why are the findings different?

99 (a) In 1990, approximately what proportion of the dietary energy intake by English adolescent children was provided by non-milk extrinsic sugars?
(b) What maximum level of non-milk extrinsic sugars intake was set for the UK by the 1991 Department of Health COMA panel on dietary reference values?
(c) What are the four biggest sources of non-milk extrinsic sugars in the diets of adolescents?

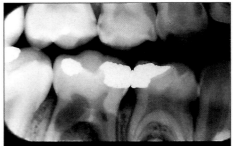

Figure 101

100 This bite-wing radiograph (*Figure 101*) was taken during a routine examination.
(a) Describe the appearance of the lower right primary second molar.
(b) What has caused this appearance?
(c) What treatment is required?

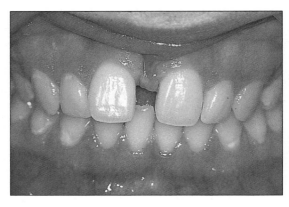

Figure 102

101 (a) What other factor, in addition to the low fleshy fraenum, has contributed to this midline diastema (*Figure 102*)? How can you tell?
(b) What will be the three main steps of treatment if the patient requests it?

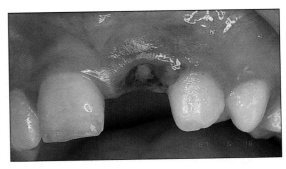

Figure 103

102 This healthy and co-operative boy with a Class I incisor relationship avulsed the left upper central incisor 45 minutes previously (*Figure 103*). The patient has the tooth in his pocket wrapped in a paper tissue.
(a) What would be your immediate management?
(b) How would you splint the tooth and for how long?
(c) What would you prescribe and recommend?
(d) What complications may be expected during the next few months?

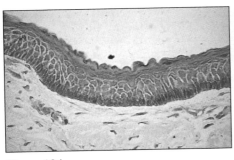

Figure 104

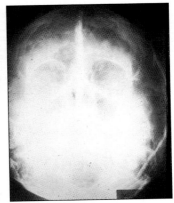

Figure 105

103 This is the lining of a cyst removed from the jaw of a child (*Figure 104*), together with an occipito-mental radiograph of the child (*Figure 105*).
(a) What type of jaw cyst is it?
(b) What does the occipito-mental view show?
(c) What would the nature of the cyst contents be?
(d) What questions would you ask to further your diagnosis?

104 What role does dietary calcium have in the prevention of dental caries?

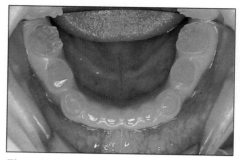

Figure 106

105 This 4-year-old boy has severe wear on his teeth (*Figure 106*).
(a) What is the diagnosis?
(b) What is the prevalence of this condition?
(c) Will there be any problems in the permanent dentition?
(d) How would you treat this patient?

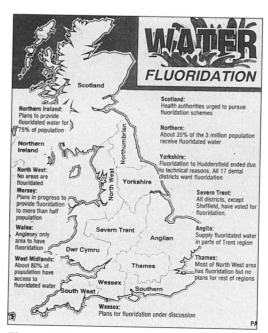

Figure 107

106 From this map it can be seen that very few areas of the United Kingdom receive fluoridated water (*Figure 107*).
(a) What proportion of the population does receive such systemic benefit?
(b) Outline the progress of water fluoridation during the 1980s in the United Kingdom.

107 This radiograph (*Figure 108*) is of an upper left permanent central incisor tooth in a 9-year-old child who attended with pain and swelling.
(a) What does the radiograph show?
(b) What treatment is required to save the tooth?

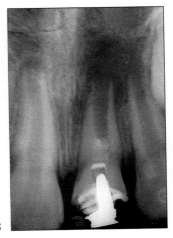

Figure 108

108 This 3-year-old child (*Figure 109*) has rampant caries of the primary dentition.
(a) What features of the distribution of the carious lesions are unusual?
(b) Suggest the possible aetiology.

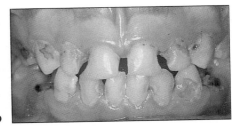

Figure 109

109 This decalcified section of a primary molar tooth, stained with picrothionin, is from a child with a history of multiple dental abscesses in the absence of caries (*Figure 110*).
(a) What histological features can be seen?
(b) What is the differential diagnosis?
(c) What is the reason for the repeated abscesses?

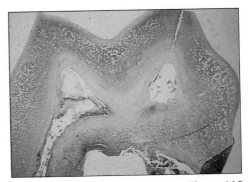

Figure 110

Figure 111

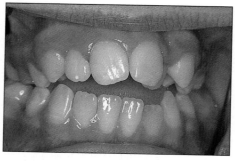

110 (a) An orthodontist decided that this girl (*Figure 111*) had endogenous atypical swallowing behaviour. What features of the clinical examination of a patient support such a diagnosis?
(b) What are the implications of an endogenous tongue-thrust for treatment planning?

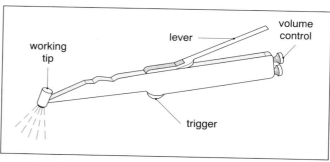

Figure 112

111 (a) What is this instrument (*Figure 112*)?
(b) How would you use it to administer a local dental anaesthetic?
(c) What problems can arise?

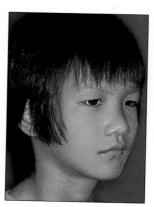

112 This 17-year-old girl has hypothyroidism (*Figure 113*).
(a) What important aspects of this deficiency influence its effects on the skeletal and dental structures?
(b) What craniofacial characteristics would you expect to observe?

Figure 113

113 (a) What is the diagnosis of this lesion (*Figure 114*)?
(b) How would you confirm this?
(c) List the precipitating factors.
(d) How could you manage this patient?

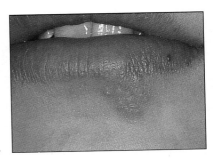

Figure 114

114 (a) Describe the abnormality shown here (*Figure 115*).
(b) What is the likely aetiology?
(c) What age was the child when this occurred?

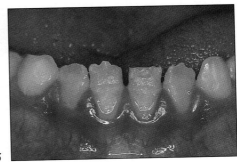

Figure 115

115 This 18-month-old child has recently had a fall and suffered trauma to her mouth.
(a) Why was the radiograph (*Figure 116*) taken?
(b) What does it show?
(c) How would you manage this patient?

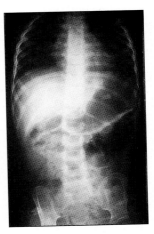

Figure 116

116 This brother and sister (*Figures 117* and *118*) had a number of relatives with clefting of lip and palate.
(a) What do you notice in these photographs?
(b) What is the significance of the family history in these cases?

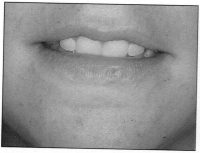

Figure 117

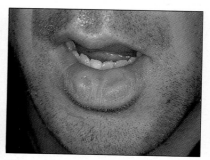

Figure 118

117 For how long should a patient complete a dental dietary record?

118 This 9-year-old boy intruded the right upper central incisor 2 weeks ago whilst on holiday (*Figure 119*) and is presenting for the first time. He is not having any problems and the tooth is firm.
(a) How would you manage this case initially?
(b) What would you do if this management was unsuccessful?
(c) What complication is the most likely to occur?

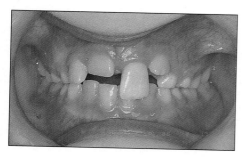

Figure 119

119 (a) What is this condition (*Figure 120*)?
(b) What embryological structures are involved?
(c) Management involves interdisciplinary co-operation between medical and dental specialities. What are these specialities and what contribution does each have to make to overall patient care?

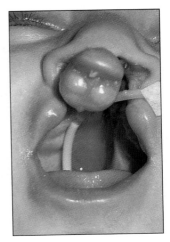

Figure 120

120 (a) What is the name of the condition affecting the lateral incisor teeth in *Figure 121*?
(b) How may such findings affect the dentition?
(c) The periapical radiograph (*Figure 122*) gives further information that will affect management of the condition; describe your treatment.

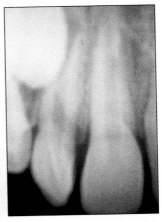

Figure 122

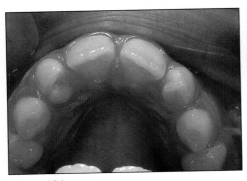

Figure 121

121 What is the difference between dietary advice and dietary counselling?

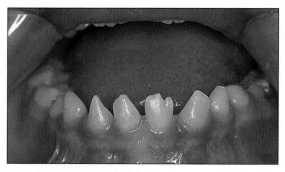

Figure 123

122 This 8-year-old girl was concerned about the appearance of her teeth (*Figure 123*). Her mother gave a history of her having skin problems. At birth she had had some linear streaks and vesicles, most pronounced on her legs but also on her trunk. These healed leaving depigmented areas but later in childhood she had developed hyperpigmented patches and streaks on her trunk and thighs.
(a) What is this condition?
(b) What is its aetiology?
(c) With what other problems may it be associated?

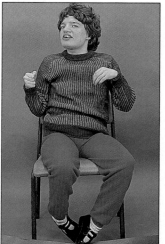

123 This young girl (*Figure 124*) has writhing movements.
(a) What condition does she have?
(b) How would you manage her dental treatment?

Figure 124

124 (a) Describe what you see on this radiograph (*Figure 125*).
(b) What is the likely scenario for what you see?
(c) What treatment would you recommend?

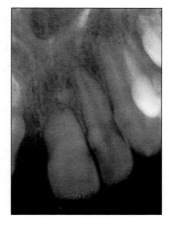

Figure 125

125 This 14-year-old Asian boy was complaining of some soreness on the inside of his cheeks (*Figure 126*).
(a) What is the diagnosis?
(b) What is the prevalence of this condition?
(c) How would you confirm your diagnosis?
(d) What is the aetiology of this condition?

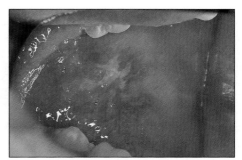

Figure 126

126 (a) Describe the anomaly in the lower incisor region shown in *Figure 127*.
(b) Are there any racial variations?

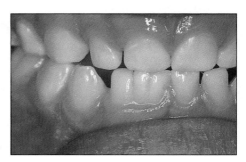

Figure 127

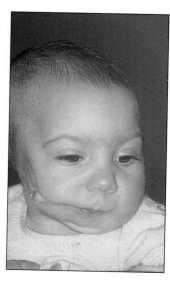

127 (a) Describe the abnormalities shown by this baby (*Figure 128*).
(b) What is the aetiology of this condition?
(c) What terms are usually applied to it?

Figure 128

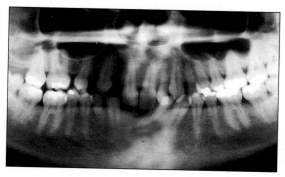

Figure 129

128 The orthopantomogram shown in *Figure 129* is of an adult female patient who has had no surgical intervention other than routine dental conservation.
(a) What is the term used to describe the dental findings?
(b) What is the differential diagnosis?
(c) What is the significance of this degree of affliction?
(d) What simple investigations can be made in the clinic to further the diagnosis?

129 What is the most commonly used scale to measure dental anxiety?

130 The lower right second primary molar in *Figure 130* is in infraocclusion; a permanent successor is present on radiograph. Assuming no orthodontic need, how would you manage this case?

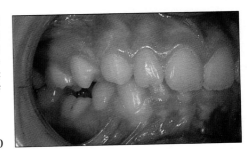

Figure 130

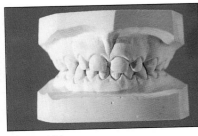

Figure 131

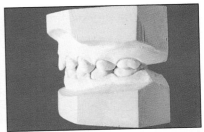

Figure 132

131 These models (*Figures 131* and *132*) display several features often considered to be ideal in the complete primary dentition around the age of 3 years. What are these features?

132 (a) What dietary factor may be responsible for the appearance of these teeth (*Figure 133*)?
(b) Outline the differential diagnosis and treatment.

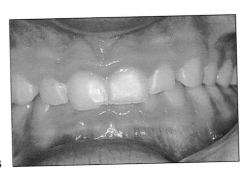

Figure 133

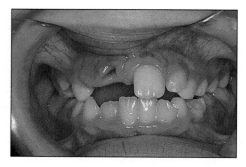

Figure 134

133 This healthy, co-operative 10-year-old girl (*Figure 134*) presented at 10.00 a.m., having avulsed the right upper central incisor at 6.00 p.m. the previous evening. The tooth has been stored in a suitable medium overnight.
(a) What would be a suitable medium?
(b) What treatment would you attempt?
(c) What warning would you give to the child and parent?

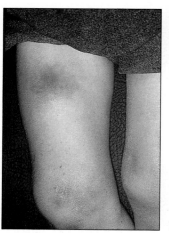

134 (a) What sort of clotting disorder does this child suffer from (*Figure 135*)?
(b) What is its mode of inheritance?
(c) How may this condition present in relation to dental treatment?
(d) How would you manage dental extractions in this child?

Figure 135

135 (a) What proportion of teenagers in the UK are highly dentally anxious?
(b) How does the dental health of highly dentally anxious teenagers compare with those who have low or moderate dental anxiety?

136 This young adult (*Figure 136*) has an autosomal recessive disorder.
(a) How has this affected his teeth?
(b) What may be done to improve the aesthetics of his dentition?

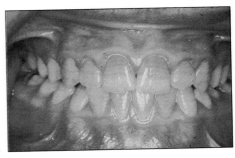

Figure 136

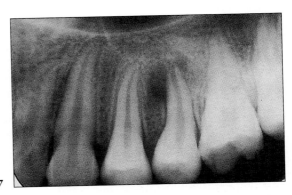

Figure 137

137 This periapical radiolucent lesion, associated with a maxillary premolar, was discovered in a healthy 15-year-old patient on routine radiographic examination (*Figure 137*). The tooth is caries-free and there is no recorded history of trauma.
(a) What is the likely cause?
(b) Describe the treatment which would be needed to conserve the tooth.
(c) What other factors would you need to consider in the management of this patient?

138 A 2-year-old child is brought to the surgery by his mother, who explains that he is fractious and has had a disturbed sleep pattern for 2–3 nights. On examination he has a flushed cheek, a circum-oral rash and is drooling, but is not pyrexic. Intra-orally he has a dark bluish swelling overlying the alveolar ridge in the upper left quadrant.
(a) What is your diagnosis?
(b) How would you treat this child?

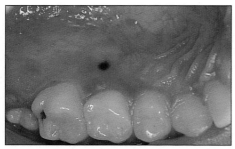

Figure 138

139 (a) Describe the lesion present on the palatal mucosa in this patient (*Figure 138*).
(b) List the causes of mucosal pigmentation.
(c) How would you manage this patient?

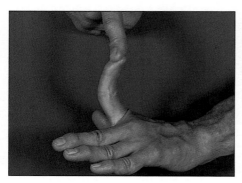

140 (a) What syndrome is this a feature of (*Figure 139*)?
(b) Why is this of interest to the dental team?
(c) What are the facial and oral signs?

Figure 139

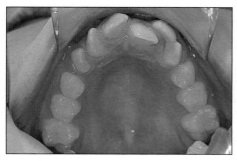

141 (a) List four types of supernumerary teeth that occur in the premaxilla.
(b) What is unusual about the maxillary dental arch of this 9-year-old boy (*Figure 140*)?
(c) What immediate treatment is needed?

Figure 140

142 (a) What do you see on this periapical radiograph (*Figure 141*)?
(b) What is the likely cause of this problem?
(c) What treatment would you recommend?

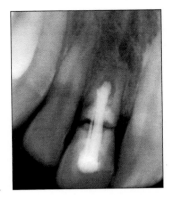

Figure 141

143 (a) With what medical conditions might the appearance of these gingivae be associated (*Figure 142*)?
(b) How would you manage this patient?

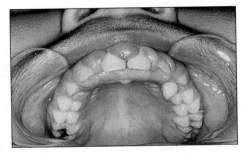

Figure 142

144 (a) Define the term 'serial extraction'.
(b) What was the originally recommended sequence of extractions?
(c) What is the objective of each stage?
(d) What are the main disadvantages of the procedure?

145 (a) What agent has produced this appearance (*Figure 143*)?
(b) What mechanism is involved?
(c) How might this patient be managed?

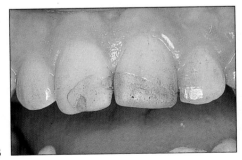

Figure 143

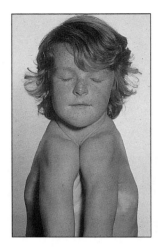

146 (a) What is this condition (*Figure 144*)?
(b) What is its mode of inheritance?
(c) What bony abnormalities are associated with the condition?
(d) What are the dental features of the condition?

Figure 144

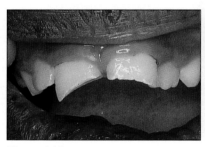

Figure 145

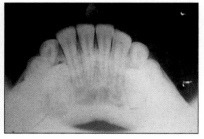

Figure 146

147 This 9-year-old boy suffered enamel dentine fractures of both upper central incisors (*Figures 145* and *146*) and the tooth fragments have not been located.
(a) What questions would you ask the boy and accompanying adult?
(b) What radiographs would you consider taking?
(c) How would you manage this case?

148 Which of the following management techniques would you think appropriate for routine dental treatment involving restorations and more than one extraction in a pre-school child.
(a) Tell-show-do?
(b) Local anaesthesia?
(c) Inhalational sedation?
(d) General anaesthetic?

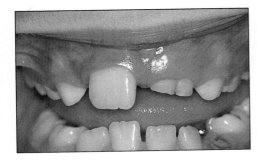

149 (a) What condition is illustrated here (*Figure 147*)?
(b) What would you expect to see on the radiograph?
(c) What treatment is required?

Figure 147

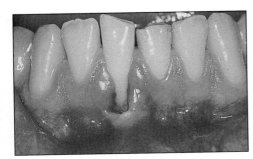

150 (a) What has produced this periodontal appearance (*Figure 148*)?
(b) What is the name of this condition?
(c) How would you manage this patient?

Figure 148

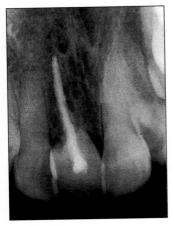

151 (a) Describe what you see on this periapical radiograph (*Figure 149*).
(b) What is the likely scenario?
(c) Is the right upper central incisor likely to be mobile?
(d) How would you manage this tooth?

Figure 149

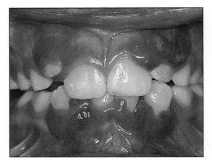

152 This 7-year-old boy had spontaneous haemorrhage from around his newly erupting teeth (*Figure 150*). What investigations would you carry out?

Figure 150

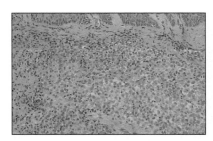

153 This histological specimen (*Figure 151*) is from the gingival biopsy carried out for the patient shown in *Figure 150*.
(a) Describe what you see.
(b) Suggest a diagnosis.

Figure 151

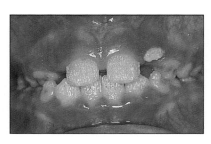

154 (a) What condition is shown here (*Figure 152*)?
(b) What is the aetiology?
(c) What is the patient likely to complain of?

Figure 152

155 Which dietary constituents are believed to be the most important in caries aetiology?

156 (a) How important is diet in the aetiology, prevention and control of periodontal disease?
(b) What nutrients are considered to be relevant?

Figure 153   **Figure 154**

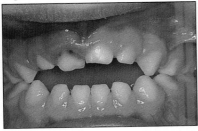

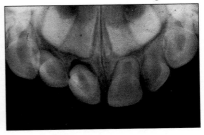

157 (a) Describe what you see in *Figures 153* and *154*.
(b) How old is the child?
(c) What treatment would you recommend?
(d) Is it likely that the permanent successors have been damaged?

158 This child was referred as she
was concerned about the appearance
of her anterior teeth (*Figure 155*).
(a) What aspects of her history
are important in establishing a
diagnosis?
(b) How would you treat these teeth?

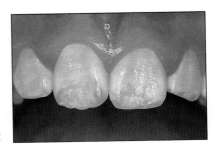

Figure 155

159 This radiograph was taken following a
fall which resulted in trauma to the anterior
teeth (*Figure 156*).
(a) What problems are associated?
(b) What treatment is necessary?

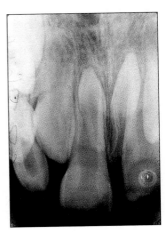

Figure 156

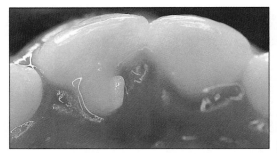

160 (a) What anomaly is present on the primary maxillary incisor in *Figure 157*?
(b) Is the succeeding tooth likely to be similarly affected?

Figure 157

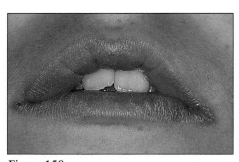

161 This 9-year-old boy is complaining of swollen and sore lips (*Figure 158*). He has a history of gastrointestinal disturbances.
(a) What investigations should be carried out?
(b) What is the probable diagnosis?
(c) How might the patient be managed?

Figure 158

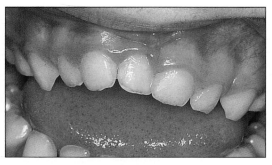

Figure 159

162 (a) What is the abnormality in the upper labial segment of this primary dentition (*Figure 159*)?
(b) What is the prevalence of this abnormality in the primary dentition?
(c) Are these teeth more common in the maxilla or the mandible?
(d) What is the mode of inheritance?

163 (a) What proportion of young children have snacks and drinks between meals?
(b) Which are the most commonly consumed types of snack and drink items in this age group and which are the most cariogenic?
(c) What substitutes would you suggest?

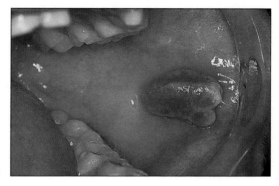

Figure 160

164 This 7-year-old patient complained of a sore lump on the inside of his cheek which bled on occasions (*Figure 160*).
(a) Give a differential diagnosis of the lesion.
(b) Suggest the aetiology.
(c) What treatment would you carry out?

165 This lateral skull radiograph (*Figure 161*) was taken to locate an anterior tooth.
(a) What does it show?
(b) What is the aetiology?
(c) What are the treatment options?

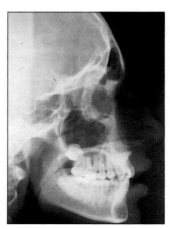

Figure 161

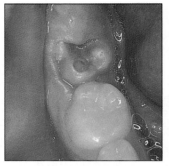

166 (a) What condition has affected the partially erupted lower first permanent molar in this 7-year-old child (*Figure 162*)?
(b) How should the tooth be treated?

Figure 162

167 Is there any evidence that edentulousness (no natural teeth) adversely affects nutritional intake and health in man?

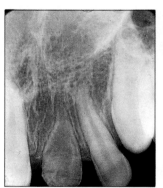

168 (a) What does this radiograph (*Figure 163*) show?
(b) What are the possible aetiological factors of this condition?

Figure 163

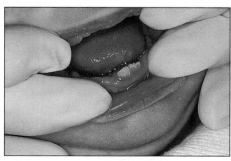

Figure 164

169 (a) What is the name given to these teeth (*Figure 164*), which have appeared 7 days after birth?
(b) Which teeth are usually involved and are they more commonly supernumeraries or part of the normal dentition?
(c) What problems can they cause?
(d) How should they be treated?

170 (a) What developmental anomaly is shown in *Figure 165*?
(b) How is the problem best treated, and what are the reasons for this approach.

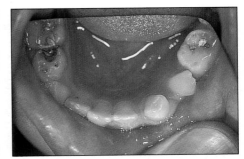

Figure 165

171 (a) What is the condition affecting this teenager's palate (*Figure 166*)?
(b) What is the cause?
(c) How is the diagnosis confirmed?
(d) What is the treatment?

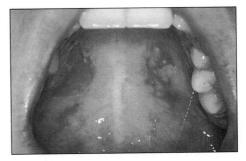

Figure 166

172 The upper left central incisor in this patient was luxated one month ago (*Figure 167*). The tooth is slightly mobile but still vital.
(a) What is the condition?
(b) What is the management?

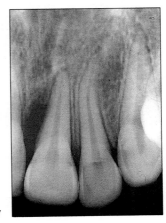

Figure 167

173 (a) How are sugars introduced into the diet at weaning?
(b) What is the significance of early introduction of dietary sugars?

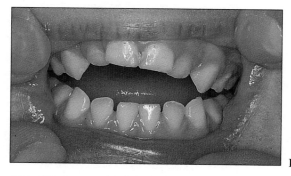

Figure 168

174 This 2-year-old child has an anterior open bite (*Figure 168*).
(a) What is the likely cause?
(b) What treatment would you advise?

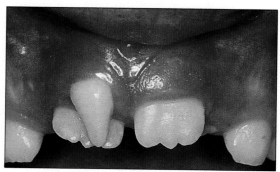

Figure 169

175 This 7-year-old girl and her parents were very concerned about the appearance of her new front teeth (*Figure 169*).
(a) Describe the appearance.
(b) What investigations would you undertake?
(c) What treatment would you advise?
(d) What difficulties might arise?

176 (a) Describe the condition of the upper right central incisor in this patient (*Figure 170*).
(b) Outline the management of this case.

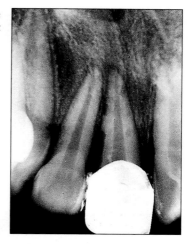

Figure 170

177 (a) What is the term given to the appearance of the mucosa in the lower labial sulcus of this patient (*Figure 171*)?
(b) What systemic condition may this be associated with?
(c) In the absence of this association, what name is usually given to the oral condition?
(d) What would histology of the oral/gingival lesions show?

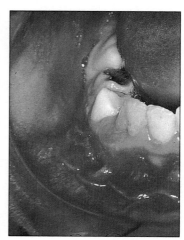

Figure 171

178 What particular dietary restrictions may patients with
(a) cystic fibrosis,
(b) phenylketonuria,
(c) diabetes
have, and how does this affect dental care?

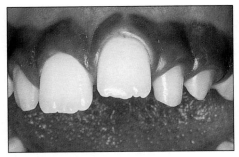

Figure 172

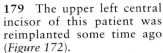
179 The upper left central incisor of this patient was reimplanted some time ago (*Figure 172*).
(a) What is the clinical condition?
(b) What is the histological process?
(c) What are the problems of allowing the situation to persist and deteriorate?

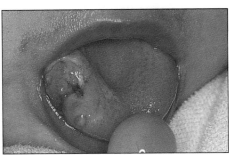

Figure 173

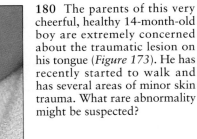
180 The parents of this very cheerful, healthy 14-month-old boy are extremely concerned about the traumatic lesion on his tongue (*Figure 173*). He has recently started to walk and has several areas of minor skin trauma. What rare abnormality might be suspected?

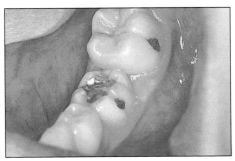

Figure 174

181 (a) What condition is illustrated in *Figure 174*?
(b) What further investigation is required?
(c) Is treatment necessary?

182 Which of the following phrases indicates low cariogenicity?
(a) low sugar
(b) no added sugar
(c) sugar-free
(d) safe for teeth (Switzerland).

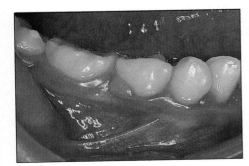

183 (a) What is the lesion associated with the lower first primary molar tooth (*Figure 175*) in this child?
(b) How would you treat this condition?

Figure 175

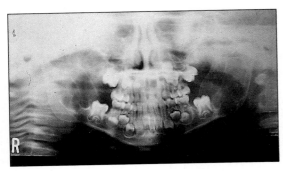

Figure 176

184 This 5-year-old child has bilateral multiloculated mandibular angle radiolucencies (*Figure 176*).
(a) What is the likely diagnosis?
(b) What is the mode of inheritance?
(c) What is the histology of this condition?
(d) What is the natural history of this condition?
(e) How is the diagnosis made?

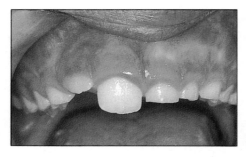

185 (a) What are the possible causes of non-eruption of the maxillary left permanent incisor (*Figure 177*)?
(b) How soon after eruption of one central should you investigate the non-appearance of the other?

Figure 177

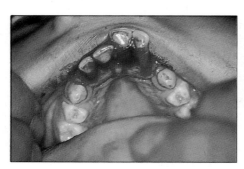

186 A 3-year-old child presented with the injuries shown in *Figure 178*.
(a) What questions would you ask the accompanying adult?
(b) What treatment is necessary?

Figure 178

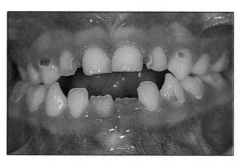

Figure 179

187 This patient's mother reported that the rampant caries was caused by medicines (*Figure 179*).
(a) Can medicines cause dental caries?
(b) Which sugars contained in medicines cause caries?
(c) How can this problem be prevented?
(d) Which alternative sweeteners are commonly used in sugar-free medicines?

188 Your local pharmacist consults you. What would you advise him to recommend to parents whose children are teething?

189 Clinically, the upper right central incisor of this patient is symptomless, slow to respond to vitality testing and firm.
(a) What does the radiograph (*Figure 180*) indicate?
(b) What is the possible cause?
(c) What is the treatment of choice?

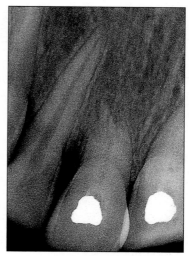

Figure 180

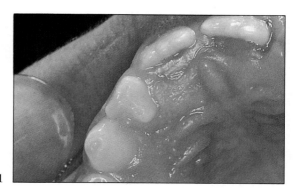

Figure 181

190 (a) What name is given to the abnormally large palatal cusp on the maxillary primary lateral incisor of this patient (*Figure 181*)?
(b) Where in the mouth do they usually occur?
(c) What is the mode of inheritance?
(d) What problems do they present?

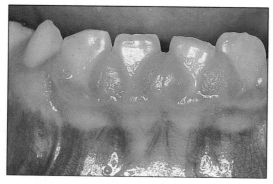

Figure 182

191 This 6-year-old boy has had a successful heart transplant.
(a) Which drugs may have caused his mandibular gingival hyperplasia (*Figure 182*)?
(b) What other drug commonly causes the condition?
(c) Why does the hyperplasia occur?

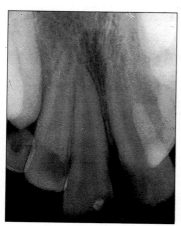

192 This patient is 12 years old.
(a) What treatment, as seen on the radiograph (*Figure 183*), was carried out on the right upper central incisor 2 years ago?
(b) Has the treatment been successful?
(c) What are the advantages of this treatment?
(d) What is the reported success rate?

Figure 183

193 What are the disadvantages of non-sugar sweeteners presently allowed for use in the United Kingdom?

194 This 8-year-old boy complained of pain in the floor of his mouth at meal times.
(a) What is the hard white lesion on the floor of his mouth (*Figure 184*)?
(b) What investigations should be considered?
(c) What treatment is required?

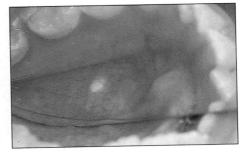

Figure 184

195 This patient's right upper central incisor has suffered a root fracture (*Figure 185*).
(a) What has been used to fabricate the splint?
(b) How long should the tooth be splinted?
(c) What has caused the staining of the splint?

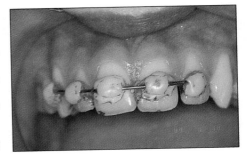

Figure 185

196 (a) What type of radiograph is shown in *Figure 186*?
(b) How old is this child?
(c) What problems can be seen?
(d) What has caused these?
(e) What treatment is required?

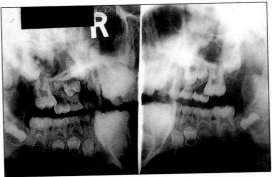

Figure 186

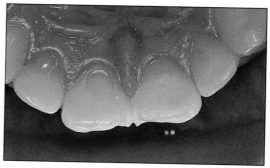

Figure 187

197 This 12-year-old girl (*Figure 187*) has cerebral palsy. She is complaining of tooth sensitivity particularly to cold food and drink.
(a) What is the likely explanation for her complaint?
(b) What is the relevance of her medical history to this condition?
(c) How would you manage the problem?

198 Does chewing gum improve dental health?

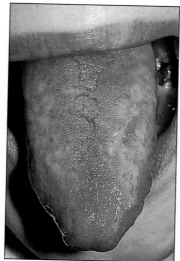

199 This 10-year-old girl attended surgery complaining of a repeatedly sore tongue (*Figure 188*).
(a) Give a differential diagnosis for this disorder.
(b) How would you confirm your diagnosis?
(c) What treatment could you suggest to alleviate the discomfort?

Figure 188

200 This healthy 12-year-old boy presented complaining of pain from his upper back teeth and general sensitivity to hot and cold substances from the remainder of his teeth. He had never attended a dentist before. The appearance of his brother's teeth was very similar.
(a) List the problems that can be identified clinically from *Figures 189* and *190*.
(b) What further investigations are required?
(c) How would you manage this patient?

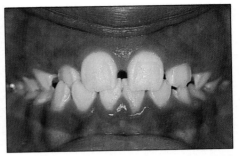

Figure 189

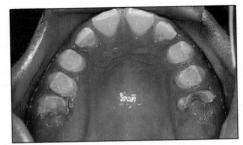

Figure 190

201 (a) What systemic condition may be suggested by the appearance shown in *Figure 191*?
(b) Detail the associated features.
(c) Does this condition have any oral implications?

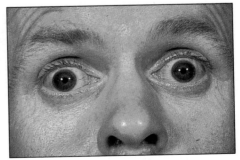

Figure 191

202 It has been shown that caries will not occur in the absence of plaque bacteria. Which species of microorganism have been particularly implicated in caries in children?

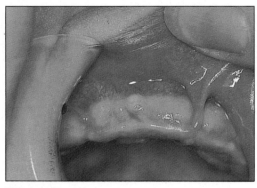

Figure 192

203 The mother of this 2-month-old baby said she was concerned about the whitish soft lumps in his mouth (*Figures 192* and *193*). They did not appear to be causing him any distress and were not tender on palpation.
(a) What are these lesions?
(b) Where else might similar lesions be found?
(c) What is their pathogenesis?
(d) What treatment is required?

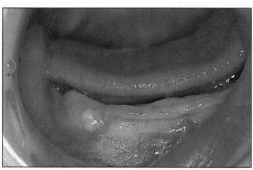

Figure 193

204 This 14-year-old girl (*Figure 194*) attended with gingival enlargement and inflammation, as well as marked halitosis. She has a large vascular lesion involving most of one side of her face. In addition, she is mentally handicapped.
(a) What is the diagnosis of her condition?
(b) What treatment might you carry out to improve her halitosis?
(c) What complications may occur?

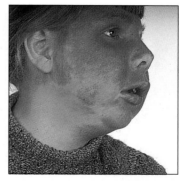

Figure 194

205 A swelling in the right upper palatal area (*Figure 195*) was noticed by this 12-year-old child. It was symptomless apart from some bleeding on toothbrushing.
(a) What is this lesion most likely to be?
(b) How should this be managed?

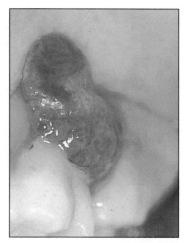

Figure 195

206 Which of the following measures would you think suitable to prevent caries in the young adolescent?
(a) Fluoride drops or tablets.
(b) Daily fluoride mouthrinses.
(c) Dietary advice to resrict consumption of sugar-containing foods and drinks.
(d) Oral hygiene instructions.
(e) Fissure sealants.

207 (a) Describe the appearance of these radiographs (*Figures 196–198*).
(b) Give a differential diagnosis.

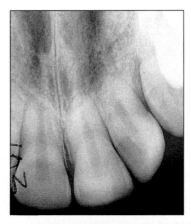

Figure 196

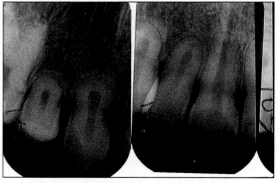

Figure 197

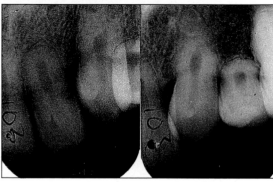

Figure 198

208 This 11-year-old child attended with a small lump on the dorsum of the tongue (*Figure 199*). This is not causing any problems except it is occasionally traumatised during eating.
(a) Why has this occurred?
(b) What would histological examination be likely to show?

Figure 199

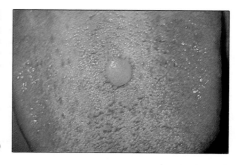

209 This young girl has marked facial asymmetry (*Figure 200*).
(a) Give a differential diagnosis.
(b) What features may be of importance in planning oral care?

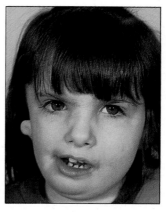

Figure 200

210 This patient attended at the age of 22 years with a swelling, tenderness and pain in relation to the upper left permanent incisor teeth (*Figure 201*). She had a history of trauma as a child.
(a) At what age did the trauma occur?
(b) What treatment is now required?
(c) How could this have been prevented?

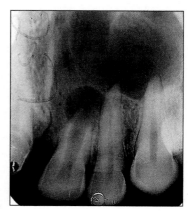

Figure 201

Figure 202

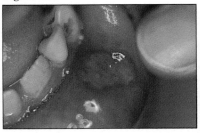

211 This child (*Figure 202*) has a history of acute lymphoblastic leukaemia. She is currently undergoing cytotoxic chemotherapy to suppress bone marrow cells.
(a) What lesion can be seen on the lip?
(b) Where and when do these usually occur?
(c) What treatment would you recommend?

212 (a) How are drug dosages calculated for children?
(b) What drug and dosage would you give to a 6-year-old child with a small atrial septal defect before carrying out any potentially septic dental procedures under a local anaesthetic?

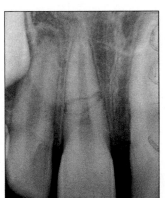

213 This child received a blow on the upper anterior teeth (*Figure 203*).
(a) What damage has been caused?
(b) What treatment is required?

Figure 203

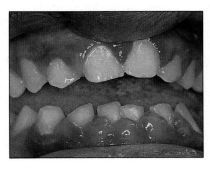

214 *Figure 204* shows the teeth of a young boy with profound visual and hearing impairment, no speech and severe learning difficulties.
(a) What is the possible cause of his handicap?
(b) What is the dental problem?
(c) How would you manage this patient?

Figure 204

ANSWERS

1 (a) The hypoplastic defect affecting the upper central incisors and the lower incisors is due to a systemic disturbance during their development, possibly measles.
(b) The upper lateral incisors commence calcification at about 10–12 months. Thus the disturbance must have occurred prior to this age.
(c) The first permanent molars.
(d) Composite tip restorations; complete veneers at this age would be undesirable.

2 (a) Finger clubbing. There is thickened tissue at the base of the nail with obliteration of the angle between the base of the nail and the adjacent skin of the finger. The nail is convex from above down as well as from side to side. Both these features combine to give the 'drumstick' appearance of the fingers.
(b) Finger clubbing is associated with conditions related to (i) respiratory system, e.g. bronchiectasis, lung abscess; (ii) cardiovascular system, e.g. cyanotic heart disease, infective endocarditis; (iii) liver and gastrointestinal tract, e.g. Crohn's disease, ulcerative colitis, coeliac disease; (iv) familial/idiopathic conditions; (v) thyrotoxicosis.

3 (a) The radiograph shows that the first permanent molar is missing. The second premolar is severely distally tilted and is potentially impacted against the second molar.
(b) This unsatisfactory alignment usually results from very early extraction of the mandibular first permanent molar, i.e. within one or two years of its eruption, particularly when the second primary molar has already been lost. The premolar may then erupt through the molar socket into the position shown. When possible the enforced extraction of a mandibular first molar should be delayed until the bifurcation of the second molar has started to calcify. This is the optimal dental age at which first permanent molar loss is most likely to be followed by good spontaneous alignment of the adjacent teeth.

4 (a) The upper left permanent central incisor is slightly less translucent than the other teeth, suggesting ankylosis following trauma.
(b) Radiography, which in this case showed a lack of periodontal space, and electric pulp testing, to which there was no response.
(c) At this stage the incisal edge could be lengthened by composite. Resorption is likely to occur and the infra-occlusion may become more severe with further growth. If extraction becomes necessary then replacement is initially by an immediate partial denture and subsequently by an etch-retained bridge. There is a danger that if extraction is delayed there will be insufficient alveolar bone to place a bridge as additional gum work may be necessary to restore the deficit.

5 (a) It is a minimal-opening Harvold activator.
(b) (i) The patient must be co-operative and well motivated. (ii) The patient must still be growing; the optimal time for treatment with a functional appliance is between 10 years and the pubertal growth spurt. (iii) Moderate to severe skeletal Class II base relationship. (iv) Mild Class II division I malocclusion. (v) Overbite normal or increased. An anterior open bite is usually a contra-indication to functional appliance therapy; (vi) No localised tooth irregularities.

(c) Proclination of the lower incisors. This is prevented by capping the lower incisors with acrylic, as shown in the figure.

6 (a) The eruption of the permanent upper right central incisor is delayed and the radiographic appearance suggests the presence of a follicular (dentigerous) cyst. This is associated with chronic periapical infection around the primary central incisor, the root of which has failed to resorb. Earlier trauma has caused loss of pulpal vitality in the primary central incisor and avulsion of the primary lateral incisor.
(b) Earlier elimination of the chronic infection in the primary incisor by pulp therapy or extraction would have prevented the development of this follicular cyst.
(c) The primary incisor should now be extracted and the lesion must be marsupialised and biopsied, with appropriate packing of the cavity. Spontaneous eruption of the incisor can be expected in a child of this age, although some form of space management may also be necessary.

7 (a) Down's syndrome, a chromosomal abnormality with three aberrations—trisomy, translocation and mosaicism.
(b) The prevalence is 1 per 600 live births in the UK. There is an age predilection, the syndrome occurring in 1 in 60 of children born to mothers over 45 years of age compared with 1 in 1000 for women of less than 30 years.
(c) Slanting of palpebral fissures
   Mid-face hypoplasia
   Tendency to Class III skeletal pattern
   Large tongue
   Teeth of abnormal shape and form
(d) Other features include:
   Mental handicap
   Hypotonia
   Short stature
   Congenital heart disease
   Epicanthic folds
   Flat occiput
   Leukaemia
   Periodontal disease
   Short hands and fingers
   High vaulted palate

8 (a) The main clinical features of 'rampant' or 'nursing bottle' caries include: (i) speed of onset—this form of caries is often very rapid in onset and the disease progresses so quickly that parents believe that the teeth erupted with the disease; (ii) surfaces and teeth affected—characteristically, the smooth labial and/or palatal surfaces of upper incisor teeth are affected, and these surfaces are normally thought to be especially resistant to carious attack; (iii) pattern of attack—with the exception of lower incisors, the teeth are most often affected in the order in which they erupt, and due to the speed at which attack occurs, there may have been extensive destruction of the whole of the primary dentition before the child presents to a dentist.
(b) The prevalence of rampant caries varies in different population groups and has been shown to change with time. Children from families in lower social classes, those from single parent families and from families where the father is unemployed have been

shown to have a higher prevalence than families in social classes I and II. Children of Asian origin, particularly those from Muslim families and from families where the parents understand little English, are also thought to be at particular risk.

9 (a) Discolouration is the commonest evidence of injury presenting in the primary dentition, accounting for 62–69% of all primary dentition trauma. Management consists of a relevant history, periapical radiographs of the affected tooth or teeth, and clinical examination. The latter should concentrate on signs of periapical infection, e.g. sinus formation. Any clinical or radiographic sign of infection is usually an indication for pulp treatment or extraction.
(b) Possible sequelae for the permanent dentition include enamel opacity/hypoplasia, root dilaceration or delayed eruption.

10 (a) A supernumerary tooth is present adjacent to the root of the unerupted permanent upper left incisor. The supernumerary is inverted and its root is completely formed, suggesting that it developed at the same time as the primary dentition. It does not appear to be causing displacement of the permanent incisors.
(b) No active intervention is needed initially and the eruption of the incisors should be reviewed. Early-developing supernumeraries often cause no displacement or eruption problems, particularly when they are inverted.
(c) In patients with protruding or crowded incisors, supernumeraries like this one may need to be removed prior to appliance therapy, even though they are not the cause of the malocclusion. Any tooth which remains unerupted may develop a follicular (dentigerous) cyst and for this reason supernumeraries which are not removed should be radiographed every 2–3 years.

11 (a) Fluorine, molybdenum, strontium and selenium.
(b) Selenium is thought to promote the formation of caries, while the other three are considered to be caries-inhibiting.
(c) The evidence for the caries-inhibitory effect of fluoride is very extensive, coming from epidemiology, clinical trials, animal experiments and laboratory studies. In contrast, the evidence for the effect on caries of the other trace elements is limited to a few epidemiological surveys and animal experiments. All are thought to have developmental (pre-eruptive) and intra-oral (post-eruptive) effects.

12 Cerebral-palsied children sometimes inadvertently traumatise soft tissues during teething. Management consists of symptomatic relief using benzydamine hydrochloride (Difflam) spray before eating. The child may also be anorexic, so maintenance of adequate fluid intake is important. Treatment and prevention of recurrence lie in fabrication of a soft occlusal splint. Impressions for this may need to be taken under a general anaesthetic.

13 (a) It is an asymmetrical anterior open bite, produced by a thumb-sucking habit.
(b) Narrowing of the upper arch due to pressure from the cheeks upon teeth that are not supported by the tongue or occlusion with the lower arch. Lateral mandibular displacement may then occur, to produce a unilateral crossbite.
(c) (i) Advise parents not to nag the child. (ii) Fit a simple upper removable appliance to cover the palate. This draws attention to the habit and reduces pleasure. If the child is below 10 years of age when the habit is discontinued, the incisal relationship may

correct spontaneously. In older children active treatment is often necessary. (iii) Expand the maxillary arch if necessary to correct a crossbite.

14 (a) Benign migratory glossitis (erythema migrans, geographic tongue). This is a common oral condition, characterised by reddened areas which change in size and shape. These areas consist of desquamated filiform papillae surrounded by an increased thickness of the intervening papillae. Histologically, there is epithelial thinning centrally in the reddened areas, with an inflammatory infiltrate mainly of polymorphonuclear leucocytes.
(b) The aetiology is unknown but a positive family history may be obtainable.
(c) This is a benign condition which may persist for years but undergo periods of remission. Only a minority complain of associated soreness. However, a blood examination should be carried out to exclude anaemia.

15 (a) The periapical radiograph shows evidence of internal resorption and external replacement resorption of 3̲ , with infra-occlusion of the tooth seen clinically.
(b) In order to produce an acceptable outcome the tooth should be extracted now. Calcium hydroxide treatment is unlikely to be successful in arresting the resorption at this stage and further loss of ridge height will make it difficult to provide an aesthetic restoration. At extraction the tooth may show signs of ankylosis (replacement resorption). An immediate denture should be fitted until healing allows the preparation of the abutment tooth/teeth for a composite retained bridge.

16 (a) (i) The report *Diet and Cardiovascular Disease* was published in 1984. (ii) The report *Dietary Sugars and Human Disease* was published in 1989. (iii) The report *Dietary Reference Values for Food Energy and Nutrients for the UK Population* was published in 1991.
(b) All three were reports of the Government's Committee on Medical Aspects of Food Policy (COMA) and were published by HMSO. They recommended that the diets of people in the UK should contain less fat (especially saturated fats) and less sugars (non-milk extrinsic sugars), and more starchy foods, fresh fruit and vegetables.

17 (a) There is insufficient space between the adjacent incisors for the provision of a crown that would be aesthetically acceptable and easy to clean.
(b) Orthodontic treatment using fixed appliances would be necessary to provide space for adequate crown construction.
(c) Space loss may have been prevented by provision of a composite restoration or a removable space maintainer soon after the occurrence of the coronal fracture.

18 (a) This figure is taken from the famous studies of Trendley Dean, carried out in the 1930s, relating the levels of fluoride in drinking water of 21 American cities to the caries experience of 12–14-year-old children in those cities.
(b) The main conclusion is that caries experience declines rapidly as water fluoride level increases from 0 to 1 ppm. This curve was important when deciding that 1 ppm F was the optimum level of fluoride in drinking water in temperate climates and the basis for artificial water fluoridation.

19 (a) A supernumerary element fused to the upper left central incisor.
(b) (i) Spacing problems in the upper arch. (ii) Occlusal problems with the lower incisors.

(iii) Caries along the line of fusion. (iv) Aesthetic problems.
(c) Division of the two elements and the removal of the smaller mesial portion. Restoration of any pulpal exposure and exposed dentine. Allowance for the mesial drift of the upper left central incisor to enable the upper left lateral incisor to erupt. Orthodontic alignment at a later stage.

20 (a) This is an eruption cyst or eruption haematoma, a bluish fluctuant swelling over an erupting tooth.
(b) A dilation of the follicular space around the crown of the erupting tooth. These usually occur in the permanent molar and incisor regions. The bluish discolouration is due to haemorrhage into the tissues.
(c) No treatment is indicated as the tooth usually erupts through the cyst. Superimposed infection occasionally requires treatment.

21 (a) By (i) visual examination; (ii) transillumination; and (iii) radiography.
(b) (i) The main method of diagnosing caries is through visual inspection. This requires a clean dry tooth surface and good lighting. Caries affecting surfaces that are not accessible to direct vision, particularly approximal caries and early caries in occlusal pits and fissures, are not easily diagnosed by this method and this is its major disadvantage. Use of a probe may aid diagnosis by helping to remove plaque, but probing early or doubtful lesions carries a high risk of damaging the enamel surface and accelerating the carious process. (ii) Transillumination is of value in aiding diagnosis of approximal caries in anterior teeth. Used in the form of a fibre optic light probe (FOTI), transillumination has also been suggested as an aid to diagnosis of approximal caries in posterior teeth. The major disadvantage of FOTI is its operator sensitivity. For reasons that are not yet fully understood, few operators have used the method with great success. (iii) Radiographs have been widely used to aid caries diagnosis. Once approximal contacts are present and the surfaces are no longer available for direct inspection, radiographs provide an important means of detecting caries at these sites. Bite-wing films provide the best information and are useful not only for approximal lesions but also as an aid to diagnosis of occlusal lesions. Many young children accept small size bite-wing films, but in those unable to do so, extra-oral films such as lateral oblique or bimolar views may be of value. Radiography has the disadvantage of requiring expensive equipment and facilities. There has also been concern about the risks involved in such use of ionizing radiation. Other methods of caries diagnosis, such as the use of dyes and of electronic caries detectors, may well be of less practical value in young children than in older individuals.

22 (a) Due to the delay in presentation and the size of the pulpal exposure, a cervical pulpotomy should be performed. After achieving local anaesthesia the pulp should be amputated at the level of the cervical constriction. When haemorrhage from the pulp has ceased, calcium hydroxide paste should be placed directly on the pulp and the access cavity sealed with polycarboxylate cement, before the tooth is restored using an acid etch composite restoration.
(b) The reported success rate for cervical pulpotomies is 95%.

23 (a) The condition exhibited by all the lower premolars is 'dens evaginatus' (evaginated odontome), in which there is an accessory tubercle projecting from the occlusal surface and containing a core of dentine, usually surrounding a narrow extension of the pulp. These tubercles may fracture leading to bacterial invasion and necrosis of the pulp followed by periapical infection, as has occurred in one premolar in the case illustrated.

(b) Yes. The condition almost always occurs in the so-called 'Oriental' racial groups and is very rare elsewhere.

(c) The abscessed premolar may be managed conservatively using a calcium hydroxide endodontic technique to induce a calcified apical barrier which facilitates root filling. The pulpal vitality of the anomalous premolars should be preserved by selective grinding to gradually remove the tubercles, followed by application of fluoride varnish on the exposed dentine. When the odontome has been reduced to the occlusal surface the tooth can be fissure-sealed. If the pulp is exposed during the reduction process it should be pulp-capped before applying a preventive resin restoration.

24 (a) Ehlers–Danlos syndrome (EDS). There are eight types (I–VIII). Inheritance can be X-linked, autosomal dominant or recessive.

(b) Cutaneous hyperextensibility
Joint hypermobility
Tissue fragility
Bruising

(c) Some patients with EDS have 'floppy mitral valve syndrome' (Barlow syndrome) or a combination of mitral and tricuspid insufficiency due to redundant chordae tendineae or valve cusps. These patients will require antibiotic cover for relevant dental procedures.

25 (a) Hypodontia (partial anodontia, oligodontia) of permanent teeth is present in 2–10% of the population. In primary teeth, hypodontia occurs in less that 1% of cases. There is often a family history of missing teeth. The teeth missing, in order of frequency, are third molars, second premolars and upper lateral incisors.

(b) Associated oral findings are microdontia, taurodontism and ankylosis of primary teeth. Other conditions in which hypodontia is a feature are ectodermal dysplasia, Down's syndrome, Ellis–van Creveld syndrome and incontinentia pigmentii.

(c) The treatment rationale is to make maximum use of any teeth present. Orthodontic tooth movement, modifying tooth contours and occluding spaces with fixed or removable prostheses are all part of the armamentarium of dental care in the permanent dentition. Implants are a viable option, as yet largely confined to those patients who have finished active growth.

26 (a) Rampant caries commonly results in extensive destruction of tooth tissue. Pulp involvement and death may occur, with consequent acute or chronic abscess formation and local and/or systemic spread of infection. Pain and swelling may not occur until a relatively late stage in the disease process. Damage to the underlying succedaneous teeth may also occur, most often as a result of long-standing infection. This may take the form of defects in enamel formation and/or mineralization, but more severe defects may also occur. In the long term, rampant caries is also thought to indicate a higher risk of caries in future years.

(b) Principles of treatment must include the relief of pain and sepsis, institution of preventive measures to arrest the disease process and, where possible, conservation of remaining sound tooth tissue. If the child is seen at a sufficiently early stage in the disease and is free of pain or symptoms, then preventive measures can be instituted immediately. Affected teeth can subsequently be conserved using conventional techniques, including not only simple restorations but also pulp treatment and stainless steel crowns, if these are necessary. If presentation is much later and tooth destruction is too extensive, multiple extractions to relieve pain and acute infection may be the treatment of choice, followed by preventive measures. Successful management both immediately and in the long term demands that treatment planning takes account of the level of co-operation of both child and parents. Medical factors may also form a major influence; if, for example, pulp treatment is contra-indicated, extractions rather than restorative treatment may be indicated for those teeth where pulp health is in doubt.

27 (a) Root maturation has continued, the apex has closed and root walls have increased in thickness due to deposition of dentine. A calcific bridge is evident at the pulpotomy site. There is no evidence of periapical pathology.
(b) No. Teeth with successful cervical pulpotomies and calcific bridges rarely respond to pulpal vitality tests.

28 (a) Extraction of these teeth is necessary.
(b) The teeth were extremely mobile and there was a significant risk of inhalation. If the teeth had not been as mobile then a soft diet could have been advised and regular follow-up of the patient. In this case the teeth would probably have become firm again. Fracture of the tooth or root is uncommon as the supporting alveolar bone is not only thin but also elastic.

29 (a) Mucous retention cyst. Mucous extravasation cyst (mucocele).
(b) Most mucoceles are caused by trauma to the duct of a minor salivary gland leading to extravasation of mucus. They are not usually lined by epithelium and, therefore, are not true cysts. The mucin-filled cystic cavity/cavities are lined by inflamed granulation tissue and infiltrated by large numbers of macrophages with vacuolated cytoplasm containing phagocytosed mucin.
(c) The lesion may resolve spontaneously but can be surgically excised with the accessory salivary gland or treated with cryosurgery. The patient and parent should be warned of possible recurrence.

30 (a) The DMFT index, where D = decayed teeth, M = missing teeth and F = filled teeth. The Index was first described by Klein *et al.* in 1938.
(b) A tooth is counted into the index only if it is decayed, missing or filled because of dental caries. The index is a record of past disease, and in older populations and in longitudinal studies suffers from 'saturation'. This occurs because once the tooth has entered one of the categories of the index, a subsequent change in its status with additional surfaces involved cannot be recorded. In addition, if a tooth has different clinical conditions presenting on different surfaces, there is no facility to record this (i.e. to 'multicode'). It may be difficult to decide if a tooth is missing because of caries or because it is unerupted, congenitally missing, or has been extracted for orthodontic purposes. Likewise with restorations, it may be difficult to determine if they are present because the tooth was traumatised or perhaps hypoplastic. Early caries is notoriously difficult to diagnose and this aspect will account for most of the variability in the components of the index.

31 (a) Dentinogenesis imperfecta.
(b) Obtain a history from the family. This is an autosomal dominant inherited condition,

although occasionally it may occur as a mutation. Radiographs show bulbous crowns with short roots and sclerosis of the pulp chamber.

(c) Restoration of the teeth with composites or crowns and the wearing of a mouth guard at night to prevent further attrition.

(d) In view of the reduced size of the pulp and consequent poor blood supply, the teeth are likely to become non-vital. This may not cause problems for years but apical infection may occur from transient bacteraemias and endodontic treatment may be impossible due to the sclerosis of the pulp chambers. In the anterior region apicectomies and retrograde root fillings may be possible, but this may be contra-indicated in view of the reduced length of the roots.

32 (a) Haemangioma–capillary type (Port wine stain).

(b) Sturge–Weber disease. The basic lesion is a congenital capillary haemangioma which involves the skin of the face and cervical areas in the trigeminal distribution, as well as the mucous membranes, meninges and choroid. It is usually unilateral. In the meninges the sluggish blood flow leads to anoxic injury in the underlying cerebral cortex which then calcifies. The clinical manifestations of this cortical damage include convulsions, mental defects and hemiparesis.

(c) If the lesion involves bone then uncontrollable haemorrhage may develop after extractions. Therefore, an intensive preventively orientated dental treatment plan is essential.

33 (a) The premolar exhibits localised enamel hypoplasia. The most likely cause is chronic periradicular infection in the preceding primary molar and/or mechanical damage to the developing premolar during the extraction of the primary molar.

(b) Chronically infected primary teeth should not be left untreated in young children. When they are extracted care should be taken to avoid damage to the underlying permanent tooth germ.

(c) The hypoplastic premolar is very suitable for a simple acid etch composite restoration.

34 (a) The right upper central incisor is immature, it has an open apex and root development is arrested when compared with the adjacent tooth.

(b) This immature tooth is non-vital. The treatment is therefore to remove the necrotic pulp and clean the root canal. Calcium hydroxide dressings are placed in the root canal at 3-monthly intervals until a calcific barrier is formed at the apex. The tooth can then be root-filled.

(c) The reported success rate for this technique is over 90%.

35 Attempt to aclimatise the patient using behavioural management techniques and inhalation sedation. She will require antibiotic cover (clindamycin, 6 mg/kg body weight) as a one-off prophylactic dose. If a general anaesthetic is necessary for all her dental care, the antibiotic chosen is 1 g of intravenous vancomycin given over at least 100 minutes, followed by 120 mg of intravenous gentamycin just before induction or 15 minutes before the procedure. She will require very intensive follow-up to reinforce oral hygiene, particularly in view of the weakness of her right arm, a result of a stroke after cardiac surgery. Chlorhexidine gel may be a useful adjunct in view of her poorly controlled gingival condition.

36 (a) (i) The change from fee per item of service to a capitation method of payment for dental care for children in the General Dental Services (October 1990). (ii) The changing role of the Community Dental Service with a change in emphasis towards caring for those with special needs and a reduction in the frequency of the screening service previously offered to children (March 1990). (iii) To a lesser degree, the recommendations in the *Report of the Expert Working Party on the Committee of Inquiry into General Anaesthesia, Sedation and Resuscitation in Dentistry* (Poswillo Report, Autumn 1990).

(b) Due to the level of funding under capitation in areas where dental caries experience is high, dental practitioners may not take on the care of these children. In addition, practices unable to offer the standard of general anaesthetic services recommended by the Poswillo Report may refer children to other centres for extractions. Preventive dental care may not be offered from dental practices, particularly for younger children. Monitoring should first take place at local level between the Family Health Service Authorities and the Dental Practice Board. Nationally, the decenial surveys of Child Dental Health give a more global picture.

37 (a) As the interval between the trauma and presentation was short and the pulpal exposure small, the tooth can be treated by pulp-capping. The exposed pulp is covered with calcium hydroxide paste, followed by a calcium hydroxide liner to cover the paste and exposed dentine. The tooth is restored with an acid-etch composite restoration to hold the dressing in place and provide a seal to ensure no bacterial contamination of the pulp under the calcium hydroxide.

(b) The reported success rate of pulp-capping has ranged from 71% to 88%.

38 (a) It is essential to establish the cause of the caries. Analysis of the diet is of the utmost importance. This child had started school at the age of 5 years and her diet had changed. She was able to obtain snacks and sweets at school which had previously been denied.

(b) Dietary advice, suggesting if snacks were necessary they should not contain sugar. The first permanent molars should be fissure-sealed. Restorations should be placed in the lower first primary molars and upper second right primary molar. During preparation of the cavities the surfaces of the adjacent molars should be inspected. The other early lesions should be carefully monitored by repeating the bite-wing radiographs in 6 months. Topical fluoride therapy would be helpful in arresting these lesions.

39 (a) Congenital epulis of the newborn. These tumours are present at birth and are more common on the maxillary gingiva. They are usually pink, non-ulcerated and pedunculated, arising on the crest of the alveolar ridge, but may be attached by a wide base. They are more common in females and in the incisor region.

(b) There is a prominent vascular component, a uniformity of structure and no demonstrable neural components. These three features help to distinguish it from the granular cell myoblastoma.

(c) Although the lesion is benign, removal under local or general anaesthesia may be necessary because it can cause feeding or respiratory problems. In reported cases excision has often been incomplete yet there has been no reported recurrence. The natural history of the lesion may, therefore, be one of regression.

40 (a) Sparse, fine hair (scalp and eyebrows)
Loss of vertical dimension (protuberant lips and chin)
Low-slung, prominent ears
Prominent supra-orbital ridges
Red face due to heat intolerance

(b) 'Ectodermal dysplasia', considered classically to be a triad of hypodontia, hypotrichosis and hypohidrosis.
(c) This syndrome is an X-linked genetic trait, the gene being carried by the female and expressed by the male. However, there are several reports of females manifesting the full syndrome and many cases of mothers exhibiting minimal expression of the gene in the form of mild hypodontia and conical teeth.
(d) Hypodontia with resultant poor development of alveolar processes. Frequent tooth malformations, usually conical in shape, and overclosure.

41 (a) It has been reported that approximately 30% of children sustain injuries to the primary dentition.
(b) A radiograph should be taken. No active treatment is required as the tooth will usually re-erupt spontaneously. However, review is required at regular intervals to check on the vitality; if there is evidence of infection, then extraction will be necessary.
(c) Advise a soft diet for a few days and give oral hygiene instruction. Warn the parents of the possibility of damage to the permanent successor.
(d) (i) Hypoplasia of crown of left upper permanent central incisor. (ii) Dilaceration. (iii) Failure of continuation of development.

42 There is white flecking present over the incisal two-thirds of the labial surface of 1 2 | 1 2 (a) Such flecking may arise from consumption of a combination of fluorides. Investigating the cause requires careful questioning of the parent about early childhood illnesses, the manner of toothpaste usage in infancy (type, amount, age at onset of use, frequency, eaten or not), water fluoride levels, other sources of systemic ingestion of fluorides in excess of the amount recommended; in this case the child had lived in an area with fluoridated water and had consumed excessive amounts of toothpaste with concentrations of 1000–1450 ppm.
(b) It is helpful to classify the appearance pre-treatment, using the Developmental Defects of Enamel Index (FDI 1992).
(c) Treatment options include the controlled acid-pumice enamel abrasion technique, bleaching and composite or porcelain veneers. (The provision of veneers could be regarded as 'over-treatment' in this case.)

43 (a) The permanent central and lateral incisors and the permanent canine are presented by hazy or 'ghostly' outlines. This is a case of 'regional odontodysplasia' (RO). This is a rare condition and, as the name suggests, is a localised disturbance of the dental tissues resulting in the typical appearances seen. The maxillary teeth of both the primary and permanent dentitions are most commonly affected. The condition must be regarded as idiopathic, although a few case reports have noted the presence of a birthmark or vascular naevus on the affected side of the face. Surgical interference with the blood supply to the jaws in experimental animals has been shown to be capable of inducing changes similar to RO, but any association with the condition in humans is as yet unproven.

(b) The condition has not been shown to have malignant potential. The rare, previously reported cases of radical resection would, therefore, seem to be totally unwarranted. The teeth make slow progress in their development but do continue to develop. The large and irregular pulp chambers preclude conventional crowning or root-canal therapy, but preformed metal crowns, followed by etch-retained restorations are of benefit in preserving the affected teeth.

44 (a) Chronological (incremental) hypoplasia.
(b) The patient was born 7 weeks prematurely and had a stormy post-natal period. The slide illustrates a chronological hypoplasia of the enamel formed during this period.
(c) The fact that the teeth are not equally affected suggests that this is not an inherited condition. The findings relate accurately to those portions of the primary teeth that were calcifying at the onset of the systemic disturbances.

45 (a) Cleidocranial dysplasia. Multiple supernumerary teeth are a common finding in this condition, together with short stature, and delay in the closure of the fontanelles and sutures of the skull. Patients may be able to approximate the points of their shoulders owing to either absence or hypoplasia of the clavicles.
(b) Eruption of the primary teeth is normal but there are severe problems with the eruption of permanent teeth, involving delay and/or total failure of eruption. This is probably associated with diminished resorption of bone and primary teeth. Recent work suggests that early diagnosis, with identification and removal of supernumerary teeth, may facilitate the eruption of the permanent dentition and reduce the need for subsequent surgical or orthodontic care.

46 (a) The right upper central incisor is infra-occluded (ankylosed) and in addition has a coronal fracture.
(b) The replanted tooth has healed by ankylosis. Adjacent alveolar bone has continued to grow normally with normal eruption of the adjacent teeth, but the ankylosed tooth has effectively ceased to erupt. It is, therefore, infra-occluded in relation to adjacent teeth.
(c) The right upper central incisor should be extracted. The root is likely to fracture during the extraction. No attempt should be made to surgically remove the retained portion which will undergo replacement resorption. An immediate space-maintaining denture is fitted prior to the later provision of an acid-etch retained bridge.
(d) A short splinting period of only 1–2 weeks is recommended because long periods of splinting are thought to favour healing by ankylosis.

47 (a) Isomalt and aspartame.
(b) Isomalt is a bulk sweetener and aspartame an intense sweetener.
(c) The following were allowed for use in the UK (in 1992):

Bulk	*Intense*
Sorbitol	Saccharine
Mannitol	Aspartame
Lactitol	Acesulfame K
Xylitol	Thaumatin
Hydrogenated glucose syrup	
Isomalt	

48 (a) Allergic contact dermatitis provoked by the metal of the appliance or one of the chemicals used in the process of bracket bonding.

(b) Delayed cell-mediated hypersensitivity.

(c) The appliance must be removed completely and the cause of the allergy investigated by patch testing using chemicals incorporated into the appliance.

49 (a) Possibly sweetened liquid oral medicines, but a more likely cause is the mother's habit of on-demand breast feeding, frequently overnight and for over 2 years. The history can be difficult to elicit as mothers sometimes feel guilty about such a practice as they are aware of the disapproval they will receive. Breast-feeding beyond a year, especially if the baby is suckled frequently overnight, can lead to this pattern of dental caries.

(b) Changing the practice can be difficult. Management includes sympathetic dietary advice. If the child is amenable, strip crowns can be placed on the upper anterior teeth and amalgam or glass-ionomer restorations on the first primary molars, since these are often also involved. Where the child is unco-operative, topical applications of fluoride varnish to the affected teeth 2–3 times a year are beneficial, together with regular toothbrushing with a fluoride toothpaste, 400–500 ppm (0.3–0.4 mg MFP), and optimal intake of systemic fluorides (fluoride water or supplements).

50 (a) Teeth present at birth are natal teeth, whereas those that erupt during the first month of life are neonatal. Despite their early eruption both neonatal and natal teeth should be considered as normal teeth that have simply erupted prematurely because they are in a superficial position.

(b) Natal teeth are seen more frequently than neonatal teeth, the ratio being approximately 3:1. The prevalence of natal teeth is estimated to be 1 in 1442.

51 The patient is at least 14 years of age, as indicated by the closed apex of the upper right lateral incisor which is root-filled. When this upper lateral incisor was root-filled, the arrested root development of the central incisor and the periapical infection had not been noticed. There was a history of trauma to this tooth at 8 years of age.

52 (a) *Soft tissues:* generalised gingivitis associated with poor oral hygiene, and exacerbated by mouth breathing; desquamative gingivitis, particularly on mucosa buccal to left upper central incisor (N.B. the patient also had skin lesions of purplish papules affecting her arms and legs, diagnosed as lichen planus). *Orthodontic problems:* anterior open bite with tongue thrust; mild crowding with retained upper primary canines displaced palatally; bilateral crossbite.

(b) Intensive oral hygiene instruction, and use of chlorhexidine mouthwash. Topical corticosteroids to control desquamative gingivitis.

53 (a) This girl has a mixed lymph-haemangioma. Intra-orally, this extends to the tonsillar area and on to the floor of the mouth on her left side.

(b) The aims of dental care should be to prevent any dental disease since extraction of carious teeth on the affected side could be life-threatening. Any restorative care should be carried out when lesions are minimal, but if the pulp is involved, pulpotomy procedures are preferable to exodontia. Fluoride supplements (1.0 mg sodium fluoride tablets) should be given daily, with instructions to allow these to dissolve slowly in the mouth. Topical fluoride applications of fluoride varnish (50 mg sodium fluoride in 1ml)

2–3 times a year are indicated if there is any evidence of dental caries either clinically or radiographically. First permanent molars should be fissure-sealed on eruption.
(c) Occasional bleeding into the mouth from toothbrush trauma may reduce the motivation for good oral hygiene measures. As the lesion extends, the airway often becomes compromised and an elective tracheostomy may be required.

54 Caries is understood to occur only when cariogenic microflora, suitable dietary substrate and a susceptible host act together over a sufficient period of time. Rampant caries has been particularly associated with dietary substrate in the form of sweet drinks given in bottles, especially when these are given at night or nap-time. Other forms of sweetened comforters, including sweet drinks in reservoir feeders and dummies dipped in a sweet substance, have also been implicated. Prolonged bottle feeding has also been particularly associated with rampant caries, as has breast feeding on demand, though rarely. *Streptococcus mutans* has been the most consistently implicated microorganism in rampant caries, usually acquired from the child's mother and becoming established once teeth erupt. Rampant caries affects relatively small numbers of children. The reason for variation in individual susceptibility is unclear, with little evidence of affected teeth having a greater intrinsic susceptibility to caries.

55 (a) This is a child in the primary dentition stage. Everything appears normal except for a root fracture of the left upper primary central incisor.
(b) Treatment of root fracture in primary incisor teeth depends upon the mobility. If the tooth is firm no treatment is indicated. If the tooth is only slightly mobile it should be left and the patient advised on a soft diet, as it is likely that the tooth will tighten up over the next one to two weeks. If the tooth is markedly mobile and is interfering with eating, or there is a possibility that it may be inhaled, the coronal portion should be removed. No attempt should be made to remove the apical portion as damage to the permanent successor may occur. The apex will undergo physiological resorption.

56 (a) Extrinsic staining.
(b) This condition is usually associated with poor oral hygiene. The green stain is produced by the effects of chromogenic bacteria in the plaque. Other causes of extrinsic staining are chlorhexidine, iron-containing medicines, drinks such as tea and coffee, highly spiced foods, betel nut chewing, smoking and heavy metal poisoning.
(c) A prophylaxis using an abrasive paste should be tried initially but this green stain may require the use of white stones to remove it effectively. Thorough oral hygiene measures should then be instituted by the patient.

57 (a) Stainless steel orthodontic wire (0.5 or 0.7 mm). This is bonded to the teeth using an acid-etch technique and material such as composite, epimine resin or methacrylate resin. The material used for the splint illustrated is a cold-curing polybutyl methacrylate (Trim). The advantage of using this material is that the splint can be simply removed using orthodontic bracket-removal pliers.
(b) The recommended splinting periods are:

Replanted tooth	1–2 weeks
Subluxed tooth	2–3 weeks
Repositioned tooth	4 weeks
Root fracture	2–3 months

58 (a) Children from groups with higher levels of caries (those from lower social classes, from single parent families or families where the father is unemployed, and children of Asian origin) may be thought to be at particular risk. Children who already have caries represent another group for whom future caries activity is thought likely to be high. Prediction on an individual basis, however, is more problematic, particularly before any disease has occurred. Those with poor oral hygiene and a high number of sugar intakes have been shown to be at greater risk in one Scandinavian study. Laboratory-based tests have been the subject of research for many years. Simplified tests of salivary buffering capacity and of the numbers of lactobacilli and *Streptococcus mutans* are now available and have been thought to be of value. However, these require quantities of saliva that may be difficult to obtain from a young child.

(b) Prediction can generally identify at-risk groups on social and demographic factors. Laboratory-based tests may be of value in identifying groups of children with existing high caries experience, but their ability to identify individuals reliably and to predict future caries activity is more contentious. Bacterial counts also have disadvantages; they are extremely variable, both between individuals and for the same individual on different occasions. Results may also be a reflection of such factors as existing caries, oral hygiene or of recent diet, rather than a prediction of future caries activity.

59 (a) Cyclic neutropaenia.

(b) There is a dramatic fall in circulating neutrophils, with a periodicity of about three weeks. The count increases again after 5–8 days but never achieves what could be termed 'normal' levels. The clear demarcation between affected and unaffected gingiva seen here is a frequent finding, but the oral lesions are more typically punched-out or apthae-like ulcerations of the gingivae, an unusual site for aphthae. The condition is genetically determined but the underlying abnormality is unknown.

60 (a) This is an invaginated odontome (dens in dente).

(b) It is often seen clinically in incisors as a palatal pit representing dens invaginatus, or radiographically as dens in dente (a tooth within a tooth). It may present as a dental abscess affecting these teeth with either caries or a history of trauma, as there is often a communication through the pit into the pulp tissue. Early use of sealants is indicated since root canal therapy is very difficult in these cases.

61 (a) The condition is called 'dentinogenesis imperfecta'.

(b) Radiography may reveal short roots, bulbous crown forms, pulpal obliteration and occasional periapical lucencies caused by attritive exposure of the pulp.

62 (a) The radiograph shows two root-fractured teeth. The right upper central incisor has been root-filled up to the fracture site. On the left central incisor there is a radiolucency associated with the fracture site. No periapical pathology is evident.

(b) In the left central incisor it is most likely that the pulp coronal to the fracture line is non-vital, while the pulp in the apical fragment is vital. The coronal pulp, up to the fracture line, should be removed and calcium hydroxide paste placed in the root canal in order to promote a calcific barrier at the fracture site. When a barrier has formed the coronal portion of the tooth can be root-filled, as in the right incisor. The apical portion does not require any treatment.

63 (a) Achondroplasia. Disordered growth mainly involves a reduced rate of qualitatively normal endochondral bone formations.
(b) This condition is inherited as an autosomal dominant trait. It is the most common of the genetic skeletal dysplasias, occurring in about 1 in 25 000 births. However, 80% of cases represent new mutations.
(c) Large head with frontal bossing and a depressed nasal bridge. Hypoplasia of the maxilla with relative mandibular prognathism. Tendency towards Class III malocclusion with anterior open bite.

64 (a) Fractured upper central incisors; gross calculus deposits; poor gingival condition, particularly in lower incisor region; hypoplastic defects on first premolars.
(b) His treatment should be carried out under general anaesthetic and this will include restoration of the upper central incisors and the hypoplastic premolars, and scaling and polishing the teeth. Root planing will also be required. The long-term dental care needs to involve his carers in carrying out effective daily oral hygiene procedures. In addition to toothbrushing, chemical plaque control measures involving chlorhexidine will be helpful. Medical advisors should be asked to check on his medication for epilepsy; this is obviously not well controlled as the trauma to his incisor teeth occurred during a fit.

65 For the majority of babies presenting with natal teeth, all that is needed is conservative management: parental reassurance, oral hygiene instruction and, if needed, alteration in feeding habits and/or the smoothing of any rough enamel edges. Babies that require a natal tooth extraction are few, and in these cases this is often due to oral ulceration of the ventral of the tongue, or occasionally to pain experienced by the mother during breast feeding. A small degree of mobility of a natal tooth should not be the main indication for its removal, since many of these teeth become more firmly established in a short period of time.

66 (a) The periapical radiograph of the right upper central incisor indicates that the root filling is inadequate and does not obturate the root canal. There are voids lateral to the root filling, which extend through the apex of the tooth. There is a periapical radiolucency.
(b) No, an apicectomy is not indicated. Apart from the technical difficulties, the child may require a general anaesthetic for this procedure.
(c) A more suitable alternative treatment would be to remove the root filling and re-root fill the tooth after calcium hydroxide paste root canal dressings have been used to produce an apical barrier.

67 (a) Fifty per cent of 5–6 year olds should be caries-free; 12-year-olds should have a DMFT no greater than 3; and 85% of the population should retain all their teeth at the age of 18.
(b) Possible reasons for the change in dental caries are:
    Increased use of fluoride toothpaste
    Changes in infant feeding practices
    Wider use of savoury (as opposed to sugary) snacks
    Falling sugar consumption
    Increased health awareness
    Improved standards of living
    Improved personal grooming

Change in oral microflora
Antibiotics in the food chain
Dental health education
Cyclical variations in disease

68 (a) The buccal mucosa overlying the apical area of the tooth should be examined for swelling or a sinus. The incisors should be examined for colour (transillumination), mobility and tenderness to percussion. A darkened crown, increased mobility or tenderness to percussion could indicate a necrotic pulp.
(b) Vitality test. Check if the pulp responds to thermal or electrical stimuli. If the tooth does not respond positively this does not necessarily indicate that the pulp is non-vital. Further evidence of non-vitality needs to be present before endodontic treatment is commenced. A periapical radiograph should also be taken and compared to the baseline for continued root development and apical pathology.

69 (a) One or more tuberculate supernumerary teeth in the line of the dental arch.
(b) The most appropriate radiographs would be an upper anterior (nasal) occlusal view and an oblique occlusal. The principle of parallax is then used to relate unerupted teeth to those that are visible in the mouth and the position of which is known with certainty.
(c) Immediate surgical removal of the supernumerary teeth and the retained primary incisors whilst the unerupted incisors still have eruptive potential. If treatment is delayed it is more likely that the apices of the unerupted incisors will close, and that it will become necessary to actively extrude the teeth using an orthodontic appliance.

70 (a) Evaginated odontome or dens evaginatus. Older names have included occlusal tubercles, tuberculated cusps, evaginated odontoma and Leung's cusps.
(b) The fracture of the tubercle exposes the pulpal tissues contained within it, resulting in subsequent necrosis of the pulp and periapical infection.
(c) The anomaly predominantly affects premolar teeth. Males are more commonly affected than females (3:2). Although isolated cases have been reported in a variety of ethnic groups, dens evaginatus is commonly seen in individuals of Chinese origin. It is estimated that 3% of Chinese children have at least one tooth affected with an evaginated odontome.

71 (a) Epidermolysis bullosa, dystrophic type. This is characterised by large, scar-producing bullae which principally affect the ankles, knees, hands, elbows and feet.
(b) Autosomal dominant or recessive. In the dominant form the conjunctiva and cornea are never affected.
(c) Development of blood-filled oral bullae after minimal trauma. These occur in about 20% of patients (like the hands in the picture), and lead to microstomia, tethering, depapillation of the tongue and obliteration of the sulci.
(d) Systemic steroids, which may help to allow some restorative dentistry.

72 (a) Fibrous dysplasia. This disease can occur in several clinical forms – monostotic as shown in this teenager, polyostotic, or as part of the Albright syndrome.
(b) Ground glass or finely stippled texture; the radiopaque area lacks an outer radiolucent zone, indicative of a fibrous capsule.
(c) Cosmetic surgical reduction, preferably when growth has stopped and the lesion is inactive.

73 (a) Was the child knocked unconscious? Is there a persistent cough? There could be the possibility that the incisor tooth has been inhaled.

(b) The buccal alveolar plate in the left upper primary incisor region is slightly expanded and there is a further possibility that the tooth has been intruded. An occlusal radiograph was taken, which verified that it had indeed been intruded.

(c) The intruded primary tooth should be left, as it is likely to re-erupt over the coming months.

74 (a) Vitamin D-resistant rickets.

(b) The radiograph shows large pulp chambers with pulpal extensions towards the amelodentinal junctions on the lateral mandibular incisor and canine.

(c) The dentine shows large calcospherites or globules of abnormally calcified dentine, separated by irregular zones of interglobular dentine. Dentine clefts in which there are inclusions of pulp tissue or bacteria are also seen.

75 (a) Hypodontia. (The term 'partial anodontia', though widely used, is incorrect.)

(b) Primary dentition 0.1–0.9%; permanent dentition 3.5–6.5%.

(c) Females:males 3:2.

76 (a) Ground section.

(b) The main mass of the tissue consists of poorly mineralised dentine matrix containing coarse and irregular tubules, and cellular and vascular inclusions. The pulp chamber is reduced in size. The enamel–dentine junction is relatively smooth and the outer layer of dentine is less disorganised than the remainder.

(c) Dentinogenesis imperfecta.

77 (a) Acute herpetic gingivostomatitis.

(b) Malaise, anorexia, irritability. Anterior cervical lymph nodes are enlarged and tender. This patient shows the inflamed gingivae as well as the characteristic coalescing vesicles on the oral mucosa and tongue.

(c) By saliva, which is heavily infected with herpes simplex virus. This is a DNA virus which, following the primary infection, is not completely eliminated from the body, but remains latent in the trigeminal ganglion and is reactivated by certain factors.

(d) There are some specific anti-viral agents available, e.g. acylcovir, but these need to be used in the very early stages of the disease. It is too late for this patient. Supportive symptomatic treatment is required here in the form of (i) anti-pyretic; (ii) high fluid intake; (iii) analgesia—systemic and topical using lignocaine viscous gel; (iv) rest; and (v) in severe cases use of systemic antibiotics to prevent secondary bacterial infections. Chlorhexidine mouthwashes will also help.

78 (a) The cement is based on the hardening reaction between aluminosilicate glass and polyacrylic acid. The acid chemically attacks the surface of glass particles, leaching metal cations out into the matrix. This insoluble metal polyacrylate contains particles of unreacted glass and fluoride complexes.

(b) (i) A unique characteristic of glass ionomer cement is that it bonds chemically with both enamel and dentine, thus reducing the necessity for extensive retention in cavity design. (ii) Biocompatability—minimal pulpal reaction, but if the cavity is deep then it is advisable to use a lining of calcium hydroxide cement. (iii) Fluoride leaching helps to prevent secondary caries.

79 (a) Lateral skull radiograph.

(b) Two shunts placed in the ventricles to drain cerebrospinal fluid (CSF) down into the peritoneum.

(c) These were placed to treat hydrocephalus. This is an enlargement of the ventricular system resulting from an imbalance between production and absorption of cerebrospinal fluid. CSF pressure is usually elevated in progressive hydrocephalus. If untreated it leads to enlargement of the head, optic atrophy, spasticity and ataxia, and a progressive decline in mental activity. The ventriculo-peritoneal shunt has a one-way valve that closes when ventricular fluid pressure falls below a fixed value.

(d) Complications of this type of shunt include bacterial colonisation, leading to recurrent episodes of septicaemia and ventriculitis. Shunt infection is less common with ventriculo-peritoneal than with ventriculo-atrial shunts. At present there is controversy over whether antibiotic prophylaxis is necessary to cover potentially septic dental procedures, but many paediatric neurosurgeons and neurologists recommend this.

80 (a) A talon cusp involving a primary incisor.

(b) Reports of talon cusps on primary teeth are increasing in the dental literature, with a high prevalence among children in India (7.7%) and Malaysia (5.2%).

(c) Children with talon cusps on either a primary or permanent tooth have also been reported to have other dental anomalies, probably due to the hyperproductivity of the dental lamina in such patients. If there is a familial tendency, therefore, it is advisable not only to examine radiographically for other dental anomalies but also to examine other siblings.

81 (a) Bilateral cleft of lip, alveolus and hard palate. The patient also has a residual fistula after reparative surgery. Another feature seen here is the impaction of maxillary first permanent molars against the second primary molars, a condition that is more commonly found in cleft palate children.

(b) The incidence of all clefts is approximately 1 in 600. Cleft lip with or without involvement of the alveolus occurs in 25% of cases and is more common in males. Unilateral and bilateral clefts of lip and palate are found in 40% and 10% of cases, respectively. Cleft palate is found in about 25% of cases.

(c) These children are usually treated by a team consisting of a plastic surgeon and/or oral surgeon, orthodontist, paediatric dentist and speech therapist. The objectives of this combined approach are (i) to achieve an aesthetically pleasing facial appearance (lip repair 6 weeks–3 months)—revisions if necessary pre-school and orthognathic surgery post-growth if required; (ii) to achieve good speech (palate closure at approximately 9 months of age and speech therapy thereafter if necessary, possibly with pharyngoplasty for some children); (iii) to achieve a good occlusion (orthodontic treatment from 6 years onwards and if necessary with bone grafting at approximately 9 years of age for some children); (iv) to provide an aggressive approach to prevention, to achieve a caries-free dentition by appropriate use of fluoride supplements where indicated, alongside dietary counselling and oral hygiene advice.

82 (a) Cerebral palsy is a non-progressive neuromuscular condition relating to brain damage in the prenatal or perinatal period.

(b) The classification is based first on the basis of the motor disorder and secondly according to the limbs involved:

Classification	Percent of cases	Physical manifestations
Spasticity	50–75	Exaggerated muscle contraction; difficulty with head control; speech, swallowing and chewing may be impaired
Athetosis	15–25	Muscles contract involuntarily, causing contorted writhing movements
Ataxia	10	Muscles respond to stimulus but cannot complete contraction that was started—disturbance in postural balance and co-ordination
Flaccidity or hypotonia	<10	
Rigidity	<10	
Mixed	5–10	

The limb involvement can be monoplegic (one limb), hemiplegic (both limbs on same side), paraplegic (lower limbs), diplegic (major involvement of lower limbs with minor involvement of uppers), quadriplegic (all four limbs) or even triplegic (3 limbs). Thus, the girl illustrated has spastic quadriplegic cerebral palsy.
(c) The implications for dental care are directly related to the severity of both the physical and the intellectual handicaps. There is a huge range of abilities and dental care needs to be managed on an individual basis. However, patients with cerebral palsy do exhibit a higher incidence of bruxism, tooth clenching, occlusal problems and difficulties with chewing and swallowing.

83 (a) There is evidence of extensive submucosal bleeding around the left upper central and lateral incisors, both of which have been displaced palatally.
(b) After obtaining good anaesthesia the subluxed incisors will need to be repositioned. This often necessitates that the teeth are first extruded slightly, their apices disengaged from the buccal plate of bone then accurately repositioned into their sockets. The teeth are then held in position, and an acid etch wire and resin splint fitted and retained in position for 4 weeks.
(c) Complications may include pulp necrosis, pulp canal obliteration or root resorption.

84 (a) Occlusal, showing the premolar teeth in plain view. The tube was not angled correctly along the long axis of the incisor roots, as indicated by the fact that these teeth are not properly in plain view.
(b) Since the angulation of the X-ray tube is not precisely as requested, the image of the buried canine crown will be projected on the film away from its true position. This may lead to errors with surgical access.
(c) (i) A long exposure time is needed unless powerful equipment is available. (ii) The main X-ray beam passes through the pituitary gland, eyes, thyroid gland and other structures. (iii) Superimposition of other structures makes the film indistinct.

85 (a) The ulceration is caused by the presence of the poorly formed natal teeth.

(b) This degree of ulceration can be intractable and lead to severe feeding difficulties at a time when it is important to establish good feeding patterns. Although smoothing the irregular tooth surfaces is a possibility, extraction of these teeth is necessary. They can easily be removed under a local anaesthetic. The child can be seated on the mother's knee and the head supported on the operator's lap. A small local anaesthetic infiltration injection should be given; the teeth can then be removed with artery forceps. Haemostasis can be established by breast or bottle feeding the baby, and the mother can provide comfort at the same time. The ulceration soon heals following the removal of the teeth.

86 (a) The primary left upper central incisor is discoloured; there is intrinsic staining which could indicate that the pulp is non-vital.

(b) A radiograph should be taken to check for the presence of apical pathology associated with this tooth. Vitality tests are unreliable in this age group.

(c) If there is no evidence of apical pathology, the tooth can be left and reviewed in a further 6 months. If there is apical pathology the left central incisor should be pulp treated or extracted to prevent the area of infection damaging the developing successor permanent tooth. If the parents are concerned about the appearance, a direct composite veneer can be placed to improve aesthetics, depending on the co-operation of the child.

87 Prevention of dental caries in the young child should include dental health education and appropriate use of fluorides. Dental health education is aimed principally at dietary modification to reduce the amount and frequency of sugar intake, and to eliminate any specific habits such as the use of sweetened comforters. Appropriate use of fluoride includes use of fluoride-containing toothpastes. Parents should brush their child's teeth for them or supervise brushing up to the age of 7 or 8 years. To reduce the risk of enamel opacities, the amount of paste should be restricted to the size of a small pea. In areas where fluoride levels in water supplies are below the optimum, fluoride supplements in the form of tablets and drops may be given and will assist in preventing caries. Recommended dosage schedules relate to the age of the child and to existing fluoride levels in the water supply. Professional fluoride applications provide little additional benefit in the normal young child who is already using fluoride toothpaste. Fluoride mouthrinsing is contra-indicated in the young child, who may well be unable to spit out effectively. For the same reason, if professional fluoride applications are to be used, fluoride varnishes carry less risk than fluoride gels. Fluoride varnishes have been shown to be as effective as gel preparations and are easier to apply.

88 (a) This boy has cystic fibrosis, an inherited condition transmitted as an autosomal recessive trait. It has an incidence of 1 in 2000, with a carrier rate in the population of 1 in 20 individuals. It arises due to a generalised dysfunction of exocrine glands. There is chronic pulmonary disease, pancreatic deficiency, abnormally high electrolyte levels in the sweat, and at times liver cirrhosis. Some salivary glands may also be involved.

(b) Finger clubbing is seen in patients with chronic respiratory disease, although its aetiology is unknown.

(c) The dental features seen here are the discolouration of first permanent molars and incisors, as well as a low prevalence of dental disease. Both of these may be related to antibiotic (tetracycline) therapy given during the period of tooth formation. Although these patients often have a high carbohydrate diet (with a large intake of non-milk extrinsic sugars to boost their calorie intake), caries rates are low, perhaps because of concurrent antibiotic therapy.

89 (a) This 5-month-old baby boy has Pierre Robin syndrome, with a cleft of his palate and a retrognathic mandible. These babies initially experience difficulties with breathing and need to be nursed in a prone position to prevent the tongue obstructing the airway. This baby is also teething, as indicated by the very reddened cheek.

(b) Causes of mental handicap may be divided into hereditary or environmental. Hereditary causes include conditions such as phenylketonuria (and other inborn errors of metabolism), microcephaly, Huntingdon's chorea, neurofibromatosis, Down's syndrome and fragile-X syndrome. Environmental causes include maternal rubella, rhesus incompatibility, viral infections and birth injury. In addition to the Pierre Robin syndrome this baby has fragile-X syndrome, which is probably the commonest cause of mental handicap, with 1 in 1500 males affected and 1 in 750 females carrying the gene for the condition. Ten per cent of all children with severe, and 6–10% of children with mild, mental retardation of unknown cause will have this syndrome. Clinical features include long faces, prominent ears, macroorchidism, hyperextensible joints and mitral valve prolapse. Oral features are large jaws, tooth wear, high arched palates and cleft palates. Behavioural changes such as autism, hyperactivity and hand biting also occur. Patients with mental handicap of unknown origin should, therefore, be investigated further for cardiac anomalies if they need invasive dental procedures.

90 (a) Intrusion or severe displacement of a primary incisor following a blow or fall.

(b) Before 2 years of age.

(c) Restoration using composite resin with the aid of a dentine bonding agent may be effective in the short term. Long-term restoration may require either a porcelain veneer or a porcelain jacket crown.

91 (a) The left upper central incisor has a vertical tooth fracture involving the crown and root. Apically, the fracture extends well below the level of the alveolar bone.

(b) In this situation extraction of the tooth is recommended.

92 (a) This is a child in the primary dentition who has suffered trauma to the upper left primary central incisor some time previously. This is obviously not of recent occurrence as there has been healing of the mucosa around the laceration. The soft tissue damage has exposed part of the root of the incisor and there is also an exposed area of sequestrating bone.

(b) (i) Take a detailed history of the trauma. (ii) Radiograph to determine extent of boney necrosis and position of permanent teeth. (iii) Warn parents of possible sequelae to permanent dentition. (iv) Extract upper left primary incisor with the sequestrating bone.

93 (a) Infected hypoplastic and dilacerated upper right central incisor.

(b) Trauma to the primary incisor at about 2 years old, possibly exarticulation or intrusion.

(c) Severely distorted crown; immature root with open apex; periapical radiolucency.

94 Not all children stand in equal need of caries preventive measures and it is important that these be used appropriately. (a) Fluoride supplements, in the form of fluoride drops or tablets, may be given to children in areas where water supplies contain less than the optimal level and are of benefit in reducing caries. They may be particularly useful in those children thought to be especially susceptible to caries, such as those children who already have rampant caries. A further group of children for whom supplements may be especially appropriate are children for whom caries or its treatment represents a greater than normal risk. This group includes children with physical, mental or emotional handicaps and children who are medically compromised. In some of these cases, where the risk of caries outweighs the risk of enamel opacities, a higher dosage of supplements has been recommended by some authors.

(b) Toothpastes are used by the vast majority of children and almost all such pastes now contain fluoride. Widespread use of fluoride toothpaste is thought to be one reason for the decline in caries seen in recent decades. This method of topical fluoride application represents an important part of prevention in the normal young child. Use of a fluoride toothpaste may, therefore, be recommended to all young child patients together with advice that parents ensure that no more than a small pea-sized amount of paste is used. Ingestion of significant amounts of toothpaste in young children may be associated with enamel opacities.

(c) Fluoride varnish applications may provide some additional benefit for high-risk children, both in those thought to be susceptible and in those likely to suffer more severely from the disease or its treatment.

(d) As with other preventive measures, dietary advice for child patients must be given appropriately if it is to be effective. Those in need of dietary restriction include children at risk of developing caries and those likely to suffer disproportionately from it. Dietary habits are related to a wide variety of social and cultural factors and may be difficult to influence. An ideal time for advice to mothers may be at weaning or before, to encourage good dietary practice from an early stage in a child's life. In giving advice to parents of young children, knowledge and understanding of the context of advice in terms of existing beliefs and habits are essential if it is to be relevant and helpful.

95 | *Indications* | *Contraindications* |
|---|---|
| Dentally anxious | Common cold |
| Marked gag reflex | Tonsillar and adenoidal enlargement |
| Traumatic procedures | |
| Sickle cell trait/anaemia | Serious pulmonary conditions |
| Bleeding disorders | Undergoing psychiatric treatment |
| Cardiac disorders | Learning difficulties |
| Physical handicap | Myasthenia gravis |
| Asthma | First trimester of pregnancy |
| Epilepsy | |
| Psychiatric disorders ⎫
Pulmonary conditions ⎭ | Check with physician |

96 The best solution will be to extract the displaced canines. The indications for this somewhat unusual procedure are as follows: (i) ectopic position of the canines so that alignment with orthodontic appliances would be difficult or impossible; (ii) lateral incisor and first premolar in contact or nearly so, so that the cusp of the first premolar is hidden; (iii) the canine is normally wider than the first premolar so that headgear support would be needed in order to provide sufficient space for alignment, further complicating orthodontic management.

97 (a) A primary double tooth, caused by fusion of the left lower primary lateral and canine teeth. In an extensive review of the literature (Brook, A.H.& Winter, G.B..

Double teeth: A retrospective study of 'geminated' and 'fused' teeth in children. *Br. Dent. J.*, 1970, **129**, 123–130.), Brook and Winter noted that the anomaly of conjoined teeth was described under a variety of titles—e.g. fusion, gemination, schizodontia, etc.— and recommended that the term of 'double teeth' be adopted.
(b) In British schoolchildren the prevalence of double teeth in the primary dentition is estimated to be 1.6% with no apparent gender preference.

98 (a) These two individuals come from families consistently affected by this conditon. The pedigree shows no male-to-male transmission. Every tooth is affected, albeit differently in the two sexes, suggesting an inherited condition. There is no other syndromic finding so these are cases of amelogenesis imperfecta.
(b) The difference of the appearances is due to 'Lyonisation', the activation of alternative X chromosomal genes (one of which obviously gives rise to full-thickness enamel whilst the other determines hypoplastic enamel) in heterozygous females. In affected males (having only one X chromosome) the only gene present is that for hypoplastic enamel. X-linked amelogenesis imperfecta has been shown to map to Xp22.2 – Xp22.3 on the short arm of the X chromosome. Most recently, a similar phenotype has been shown to map to a site on the long arm of the X.

99 (a) In 1990 about 17% of dietary energy intake by English adolescents was provided by non-milk extrinsic sugars; total sugars provided about 22% of energy intake.
(b) The 1991 COMA panel recommended that the intake of non-milk extrinsic sugars by the UK population should be: minimum = 0%; maximum 10% of total energy intake or 11% of food energy intake (the latter excludes alcohol intake).
(c) The four biggest sources of non-milk extrinsic sugars are: confectionery, soft drinks, table sugars, biscuits and cakes—these provide over 80% of non-milk extrinsic sugars intake.

100 (a) This tooth has been restored with amalgam. The mesio-occlusal restoration appears to be closely related to the pulp. There is an intra-radicular area of radiolucency and extensive internal resorption of the radicular and coronal pulp.
(b) The pulp has become necrotic, due either to the original carious lesion or to the placement of the restoration. Both the internal resorption and the inter-radicular radiolucency are due to pulpal inflammation and necrosis.
(c) The internal resorption is too extensive to permit adequate endodontic therapy. The tooth should, therefore, be extracted.

101 (a) The maxillary incisors are small in relation to the mandibular ones. This is indicated by the fact that the canine relationship is Class I and the overjet is normal.
(b) (i) Fraenectomy. (ii) Approximation of incisors using a fixed appliance to maintain axial inclinations. (iii) Building up crown sizes with composite resin or crowns to close spaces and prevent relapse.

102 (a) The tooth should be examined and, if it is not damaged, placed in physiological saline whilst the history and examination is conducted. The tooth should be replanted after achieving good local anaesthesia.
(b) The tooth can be splinted using acid-etch resin and wire splint, which will allow slight movement of the replanted tooth. The tooth should be splinted for 1–2 weeks.
(c) A five-day course of antibiotics should be prescribed. Chlorhexidine mouth wash

should be used twice daily to aid plaque control. The patient's anti-tetanus status must be checked, and if there is any doubt he should be referred to his general medical practitioner. Advice should be given on a soft diet and fluid intake.

(d) For avulsed teeth with open apices which are replanted immediately after the accident, there is the possibility that the pulp will revascularise but it is unlikely in this case. Treatment using a non-setting $Ca(OH)_2$ will, therefore, be required. A further complication is that the tooth might undergo root resorption. The parents should be advised of the possible sequelae following replantation.

103 (a) The cyst is an odontogenic keratocyst.

(b) The occipito-mental radiograph shows calcification of the falx cerebri and meninges.

(c) Clinical aspiration of the cyst could aid diagnosis by revealing a thick, creamy fluid, without the smell of pus. A stained smear of this aspirate would show the presence of desquamated keratin. The level of soluble protein would be low.

(d) This is a case of basal cell naevus syndrome (Gorlin's syndrome). Enquiries should be made as to whether other family members are similarly affected or whether there is a history of pigmented skin lesions (basal cell naevi). Keratocysts have been reported in the age range 1–80+ years. Examination should also include possible rib anomalies, fused vertebrae and frontal or parietal bossing of the skull. Regular investigation at periods of about 6 months has been strongly recommended to detect newly arisen skin or jaw lesions at the earliest opportunity.

104 The role of dietary calcium in protection against dental caries is still unclear. Because teeth consist largely of calcium and phosphorus, dietary calcium would be expected to be protective. Pre-eruptively, however, vitamin D is likely to be of greater importance than calcium. Sometimes it is difficult to decide whether a dietary effect is pre-eruptive or post-eruptive, as in the case of the protective effect of hard water (although calcium in water is much less important than fluoride). Post-eruptively, the caries-protective effect of cheese may be due in part to raised levels of calcium in the saliva and plaque. However, chewing gums, sweets and breakfast cereals fortified with calcium has little effect on human caries, and any effect is more likely to be due to raised phosphate levels.

105 (a) Dentinogenesis imperfecta.

(b) Approximately 1 in every 8000 people are affected, but there is considerable variation in expression, ranging from a very mild discolouration to the severe form shown here.

(c) Both dentitions will be affected.

(d) There was such severe attrition that both aesthetics and function were compromised. Over-dentures were, therefore, constructed for this patient. Full preventive care and advice were given.

106 (a) Twelve per cent of the UK population receive fluoridated water (10% artificially, 2% naturally fluoridated).

(b) 1983: Lord Jauncey pronounced on the Strathclyde case. Outcome: fluoridation of the water supply not legal in Scotland; 1985: Water Fluoridation Act, enabling legislation to permit fluoridation in areas where Health Authorities request it; 1988: Dispute between the Water Authorities Association and the Department of Health over indemnity for any accident arising from fluoridation; 1989: Department of Health agree to 100% indemnity cover; 1991: Water Industries Act, renaming of 1985 Water Fluoridation Act.

107 (a) There is extensive loss of coronal tissue which has had some form of post restoration placed. The apex is immature, suggesting that the injury took place about a year to 18 months previously. There is extensive apical radiolucency as a result of infection. It would seem that a pulpotomy was performed.
(b) If drainage cannot be obtained by removal of the crown and access to the root canal, a five-day course of antibiotics should be commenced plus hot salt mouthwashes. When the infection has been eliminated, a dressing of calcium hydroxide should be placed to induce apical closure and prepare the canal for root filling. When a sufficient apical barrier has been achieved a permanent root filling and coronal restoration may be placed.

108 (a) Although the caries is very widespread it does not conform to the distribution seen from frequent intake of sugary liquids from a comforter bottle used particularly at night. This leads to cervical lesions, notably in the maxillary incisors. The patient illustrated here shows approximal lesions in both upper and lower incisors, as well as in the primary molars. The lower incisors are usually relatively protected from the effects of sugary substances in a bottle or dummy by the pooling of the saliva in this area, and by the position of the tongue covering these teeth during suckling.
(b) The aetiology is related to sucrose consumption in an adhesive form rather than in a liquid form from a bottle. The mother had conscientiously applied dietary restrictions to sweets and sugary snacks, but the child had been on long-term sucrose-based medication for epilepsy.

109 (a) The section shows physiological attrition, interglobular dentine, elongation of the pulp horns and pulp necrosis.
(b) The differential diagnosis should include both vitamin D-dependent and vitamin D-resistant rickets. Up to 30% of cases of rickets may present because of dental findings. There may also be delayed eruption of teeth, and an absent or poorly defined lamina dura. It has been suggested that gross enamel hypoplasia is more often associated with the resistant form of the disease.
(c) The abscesses result from exposure of the elongated pulp cornuae following minimal tooth tissue loss due to attrition, abrasion and erosion.

110 (a) (i) A tongue that is particularly acute and visible during speech and swallowing. (ii) Anterior open bite. (iii) Proclination of maxillary, and mandibular, incisors, although the lowers may be retroclined by the action of the lower lip. (iv) A lisp.
(b) Endogenous tongue thrust is a normal neuromuscular rather than adaptive or habitual activity. It is not modified if tooth positions are changed so that overjet reduction will relapse under its influence. Orthodontic treatment must therefore be limited to aligning teeth within the arches in which they are placed and not attempting to alter the overjet.

111 (a) A 'jet syringe'. Earlier versions of the jet syringe were the 'Dermajet' followed by the 'Panjet' and 'Syrijet'. However, nearly three decades of clinical studies have not conclusively shown the jet syringe to be as effective as, or to have major advantages over, the conventional syringe. This is due primarily to the limited depth of penetration

achieved by the anaesthetic solution, resulting in unreliable anaesthesia.
(b) A jet of local anaesthetic is administered through the mucosa.
(c) More bleeding, pain and post-operative bruising are commonly experienced following the jet injection technique over and above a conventional syringe injection.

112 (a) Hypothyroidism can be either congenital or acquired. Clinical manifestations depend on the age of onset, the extent of the dysfunction and the length of time before the condition is effectively treated. If the thyroid deficiency is not rectified for a long period, skeletal maturity and dental development are affected. Skeletal maturity is more retarded than dental development. Following adequate treatment the skeletal maturity improves more quickly whilst the dental development is less responsive.
(b) Craniofacial growth is affected by retardation in velocity rather than by modification in its pattern. There is a tendency for small facial height and an open anterior bite. A high caries experience is commonly observed and, although there is no characteristic alteration in morphology, enamel defects are common.

113 (a) Herpes labialis.
(b) Viral swabs of the lesion should be taken and sent for culture of herpes simplex virus on baby hamster kidney (BHK) cells or occasionally electron microscopy. Serology is *not* of value here.
(c) (i) Common cold (upper respiratory tract infections). (ii) Ultra-violet light. (iii) Mechanical trauma. (iv) Stress. (v) Menstruation. (vi) Depressed cell mediated immunity.
(d) Acyclovir cream (5%) may reduce the duration, if applied topically (every four hours for five days) during the prodromal phase. The patient should be advised as to the contagious nature of the lesions.

114 (a) There is a band of hypoplasia affecting the lower permanent incisor teeth. This is known as 'chronological' or 'incremental' hypoplasia.
(b) A systemic disturbance affecting the formation of the enamel matrix. Over 100 factors have been reported to cause hypoplastic defects, but the most common are the exanthematous diseases such as measles and nutritional disorders.
(c) The lower permanent incisor teeth commence calcification at approximately 3–4 months after birth. There is a small amount of normal enamel just on the incisal edges of these teeth followed by a broad band of hypoplasia. This boy was introduced to mixed feeding from the age of 5 months and then failed to thrive. He was diagnosed after some months as having Coeliac disease (gluten sensitive enteropathy), a sensitivity of the small intestine to gluten in wheat and other cereals. Once established on a gluten-free diet the symptoms resolved and the remaining part of the enamel has developed and calcified normally. Thus, the hypoplastic defects developed between 5–18 months of age.

115 (a) The child had suffered extensive intra-oral trauma; the left upper primary incisor tooth appeared to be missing and could not be found at the site of the accident. Intra-oral radiographs confirmed that the tooth had not been intruded. This chest X-ray was taken, therefore, to see whether the tooth had been swallowed or inhaled.
(b) The tooth is visible in the stomach. It is important to have an expert radiological opinion as it is sometimes difficult to be sure whether foreign bodies are situated in the stomach or lungs.
(c) The parents and child should be reassured. A high-bulk diet should encourage the

tooth to pass through the gastro-intestinal tract uneventfully. It is wise to check the faeces to confirm this.

116 (a) These are examples of 'van der Woude syndrome', showing lip-pits unilaterally in the female and bilaterally in the male.
(b) This is an autosomal dominant trait involving cleft lip and/or cleft palate occurring in association with lower lip pits or elevations. The condition shows very variable expression and these individuals may in their turn have offspring with more or less marked stigmata.

117 When a comprehensive analysis of a patient's diet is required for dental purposes, a three-day record should be obtained. The length of time a diet record should be completed depends on the items under examination, so if an individual's carbohydrate, fat and vitamin intake is under examination, a seven-day diet record would be needed. However, with regard to dental health, dietary records are commonly used in the prevention of dental caries and erosion of tooth tissue. Therefore, since it is the amount and frequency of sugar and/or the consumption of acidic foods and beverages that are under assessment, a three-day record is sufficient. This is because sugar and acidic drinks are consumed fairly regularly throughout the week and little extra information is gained after three days have been documented. One of the three days should be on a weekend.

118 (a) A detailed examination should be conducted which will include vitality testing of all incisor teeth and periapical radiographs to act as baseline for future reviews. The clinical crown height of the right upper central incisor should be measured together with the level of the incisal plane between the central incisors. The intruded incisor does not require any active treatment at the moment as it may re-erupt.
(b) The patient should be reviewed after 3 months and the clinical crown height of the intruded tooth checked, together with the level of the incisal plane. If the tooth has not shown any re-eruption the tooth will need to be extruded orthodontically.
(c) The patient needs to be reviewed regularly as there is a high risk of pulp necrosis and root resorption following an intrusion injury.

119 (a) A complete bilateral cleft of lip and palate.
(b) This type of cleft involves failure of fusion between the frontonasal and maxillary processes in the primary palate and between the palatal shelves of the secondary palate.
(c) (i) The orthodontist provides a feeding plate to help during the neonatal period. Occlusal anomalies are frequently associated with a cleft and the orthodontist is again involved in aligning the developing dentition and preparing the teeth to stabilise a bone graft. (ii) The general dental practitioner provides whole mouth preventive care to maintain the dentition. (iii) The paediatric surgeon repairs the tissue defect to restore appearance and function. (iv) The ENT surgeon may fit grommets or T tubes to minimise recurrent middle ear infections. (v) The speech therapist assists with phonation problems.

120 (a) These odontomes are sometimes given the name 'talon cusps' since they resemble the talons of a bird of prey.
(b) They may cause labial displacement of the incisor teeth and they may permit caries to form in the cleft between the talon and the rest of the tooth.

(c) The radiograph shows an additional pulp filament extending into the talon cusp. The tooth is being displaced and, therefore, the talon requires progressive reduction over a considerable period to permit deposition of secondary dentine.

121 Dietary advice merely imparts information. It fails to relate the dietary information to the patient's individual circumstances or lifestyle. Dietary advice, by providing little feedback, does not allow any opportunity to correct misunderstandings or to give positive reinforcement when the messages are understood. Examples of methods used in giving such advice are audiovisual aids, printed literature and verbal presentation. Dietary counselling, on the other hand, obtains a personal record of the patient's own dietary pattern and counsels the patient using this information. Such counselling is therefore based on the patient's personal lifestyle and is of direct relevance to the individual. This enhances the possibility of the patient's compliance with the clinician's recommendations.

122 (a) Incontinentia pigmenti (Bloch–Sulzberger syndrome).
(b) It is a rare inherited multisystem disorder thought to be transmitted as an X-linked dominant trait. The mutated gene is usually lethal *in utero* for males, thus females are almost exclusively affected.
(c) The skin lesions may be the only manifestation but about 80% of affected children have other defects. Over half have dental anomalies consisting of hypodontia, conical and malformed teeth and delayed eruption. Alopecia occurs in up to 40%. CNS manifestations including developmental retardation, epilepsy, microcephaly, spasticity and paralysis are found in about one-third of affected individuals.

123 (a) She has the athetoid form of cerebral palsy.
(b) A limited amount of treatment may be possible such as a scale and prophylaxis and restorations in the anterior region. Appointments should be kept short. More extensive treatment may necessitate a general anaesthetic under 'day stay' conditions.

124 (a) The root canal of the left upper central incisor is obliterated and the tooth has a very broad rounded apex. The root of this tooth is shortened in comparison with the adjacent tooth. There is an apical fragment present, well separated from the coronal part of the tooth. The right central incisor has been avulsed and not replanted.
(b) The left upper central incisor suffered a root fracture several years ago, which did not heal by calcific union. As this tooth erupted the apex was left behind in the alveolus. As part of the healing process the fractured surface of the root became rounded and the apex has started to resorb. As a complication of healing there has been root canal obliteration.
(c) The tooth has remained vital and there is no pathology; therefore, no treatment is recommended. The patient should be advised of the short root and prognosis in the event of further trauma.

125 (a) Lichen planus.
(b) The prevalence in the general population is approximately 1%. It is, however, rare in children but there are no accurate data. There is a slight female predominance and a greater prevalence in people of Asian origin.

(c) Lichen planus is usually diagnosed from its clinical features and the involvement of skin and other mucous membranes. The characteristic skin lesions are flat-topped violaceous papules about 2–4 mm in diameter. These predominantly affect the lumbar regions, flexor surfaces of the wrists and anterior surface of the lower limbs. However, the condition can closely simulate lupus erythematosus and biopsy may be indicated. The histopathological features include:
(i) 'Saw tooth' rete ridges.
(ii) Hyperorthokeratosis or hyperparakeratosis.
(iii) Thickening of granular cell layer.
(iv) Basal cell liquefaction.
(v) Dense, band-like inflammatory cell infiltrate in the upper lamina propria.
(d) The aetiology is usually unknown, but in some patients various drugs or dental restorative materials have been identified. It may be associated with various systemic disorders such as diabetes, but the majority of patients with lichen planus are otherwise well.

126 (a) This is an example of a conjoined tooth. The lower right primary central incisor appears to be geminated and then fused to the lateral incisor. Gemination is an abortive attempt by a single tooth bud to divide and is due to the invagination of the developing dental organ. Fusion is the embryologic union of normally discrete organs. If it occurs early, the two developing teeth will unite to form a single tooth of almost normal size. However, if it occurs very late, one tooth almost twice the normal size will develop, possibly with a notch in the incisal edge. In this particular case both gemination and fusion appear to have occurred—unless the possibility of a supernumerary tooth being part of the fusion process is considered!
(b) Racial variations are seen: a 5% prevalence of fusion has been reported in a Japanese population compared with 0.5% figure in several Caucasian populations.

127 (a) This is a unilateral condition with marked facial asymmetry due to abnormalities and displacement of the ear and underlying abnormalities of facial support. The maxillary, temporal and malar bones are reduced in size and flattened. There is gross hypoplasia of the mandibular ramus and condyle. The ear appears to be a small, ill-defined mass of tissue displaced anteriorly and inferiorly.
(b) Most cases are sporadic and believed to be due to haemorrhage and expanding haematoma formation in the embryological stapedial artery complex. The anomalies suggest their origin at about 30–45 days' gestation.
(c) Oculo-auriculo vertebral spectrum; hemifacial microsomia; first branchial arch syndrome; Goldenhar syndrome; first and second branchial arch syndrome; unilateral mandibulofacial dysostosis, etc.

128 (a) Hypodontia (anodontia is a complete absence of teeth, oligodontia may be used to describe the absence of more than half the teeth, partial anodontia is a nonsense term). Tooth size is frequently reduced and the maximum convexity of the tooth crowns is apically displaced, which may be of significance when designing prostheses. There is a characteristic increase in molar pulp size.
(b) Genetic factors including familial hypodontia (most commonly), ectodermal dysplasia, Down's syndrome; local factors including trauma, ionising radiation, jaw

fracture, hormonal influences and metabolic imbalance. Osteomyelitis would be unlikely to produce a symmetrical appearance.

(c) Hypodontia affecting more than four teeth is much more likely to be associated with systemic conditions. The diagnosis here is the X-linked form of hypohidrotic ectodermal dysplasia. Whilst females show mild to moderate stigmata of the condition, affected males may die in infancy from undiagnosed hyperthermia.

(d) This uncommon condition affects tissues of ectodermal origin, including hair, teeth and sweat glands. The most profitable investigation is to establish the family history; severely affected males, no male-to-male transmission and a history of stillbirths or male infant deaths are indicative of X-linked hypohidrotic ectodermal dysplasia. All findings are markedly more pronounced in affected males than carrier females. Enquiry as to whether the patient can tolerate hot weather, together with examination of the hair (which is fine and sparse even in 'carrier', i.e. heterozygous, females) and fingers (which may show the absence or reduction of sweat pores, detectable either by the naked eye or by a sense of 'dry hands'), further support the diagnosis. Definitive diagnosis is by referral to a clinical geneticist who will carry out tests for sweat functions, together with molecular biological investigations.

129 The Corah Dental Anxiety Scale (CDAS). This is a well-established index, measuring reactions on a five-point scale of ascending anxiety to four different dental treatment situations: before attending the dental surgery, waiting in the dental surgery, sitting on the dental chair, having treatment. The maximum CDAS score, therefore, is 20. A score of 15 or more is a strong indication of high dental anxiety.

The Corah Dental Anxiety Scale

Tick the answer that best describes your feelings:

1 If you had to go to the dentist tomorrow, how would you feel about it?
  I would look forward to it as a reasonably enjoyable experience.
  I wouldn't care one way or the other.
  I would be a little uneasy about it.
  I would be afraid that it would be unpleasant and painful.
  I would be very frightened of what the dentist might do.

2 When you are waiting in the dentist's surgery for your turn in the chair, how do you feel?
  Relaxed.
  A little uneasy.
  Tense.
  Anxious.
  So anxious that I sometimes break out in a sweat and feel physically sick.

3 When you are in the dentist's chair waiting while he gets his drill ready to begin working on your teeth, how do you feel?
  Relaxed.
  A little uneasy.
  Tense.
  Anxious.
  So anxious that I sometimes break out in a sweat and feel physically sick.

4 You are in the dentist's chair waiting to have your teeth cleaned. While you are waiting and the dentist is getting out the instruments which he will use to scrape your teeth around the gums, how do you feel?

Relaxed.
A little uneasy.
Tense.
Anxious.
So anxious that I sometimes break out in a sweat and feel physically sick.

130 In general, retained primary molar teeth are eventually shed and have no long-term effect on occlusal development. However, individual cases may prove the exception to this and a regular, rigorous pattern of follow-up is recommended.

131 (i) Spacing between the incisors. (ii) The incisors are upright and the overbite is increased. (iii) Anthropoid spaces, mesial to the upper primary canine and distal to the lower primary canine. (iv) A flush terminal plane on the second primary molars.

132 (a) Erosion from acidic compounds in the diet has removed dental enamel, creating a flattening of the labial surfaces of maxillary incisor teeth.
(b) Post-eruptive tooth wear needs to be distinguished from pre-eruptive enamel hypoplasias—the latter are usually rough, while tooth wear results in smooth tooth surfaces. The three causes of tooth wear are erosion, attrition and abrasion. These are usually seen in combination; for example, erosion of free smooth surfaces may well be accelerated by toothbrush abrasion, and erosion of occlusal surfaces may be accelerated by attrition. It is important to spot erosion early, identify the cause and eliminate it if possible; otherwise, replacement of tooth tissue for cosmetic or other purposes can be difficult and expensive.

133 (a) Physiological saline is a recommended storage medium. However, this is not usually available as a first aid measure at the site of the accident. Milk is a suitable storage medium and is usually readily available.
(b) Even though the tooth has been out of the mouth for 16 hours, it is still worth attempting to replant. Teeth have been successfully replanted up to 24 hours after being avulsed.
(c) The child and parent should be warned that the prognosis is poor. It is likely that the tooth will undergo root resorption. The tooth may remain in place for only a few months or may remain as an excellent space maintainer throughout the remaining period of dento-facial growth.

134 (a) Coagulation defect, in this case haemophilia A. The condition is characterised by deep bleeding into muscles and joints.
(b) X-linked recessive; 1 in 10 000 males are affected.
(c) Bleeding time may be normal but clotting is grossly impaired, so there is typically a delayed onset of persistent bleeding after injury (e.g. extraction). Trauma (including local anaesthetic injections) causes deep soft-tissue bleeding and haematoma formation.
(d) (i) Carry out pre-operative radiographic dental assessment. (ii) Admit the patient to hospital; (iii)Give adequate clotting factor replacement, plus an anti-fibrinolytic agent (EACA or tranexamic acid). (iv) Give local analgesia, but avoid dental block injections (use intraligamentary and infiltration analgesia). (v) Extract the tooth. (vi) Suture the

socket and place haemostatic foam in the socket. (vii) Keep under observation—more factor replacement may be necessary. (viii) Give analgesia (*not* aspirin).

135 (a) The prevalence of high dental anxiety among teenagers is approximately 7–14%.

(b) In general, dentally anxious **teenagers** have a higher dental caries experience (DMFT) than their contemporaries. In particular, they have more missing teeth and have less teeth fissure-sealed. They also, when compared with children with low or moderate dental anxiety, are more likely to:
• cancel an appointment because of fear
• have had their last dental visit more than one year ago
• have last visited a dentist for reasons other than a 'check-up'
• brush their teeth less frequently than once per day
• spend more money on sweets per day
• consume carbonated sugary drinks more frequently.
On the whole, children with a high dental anxiety do not help themselves by adopting a more positive attitude to the prevention of disease in their own mouths.

136 (a) The condition is cystic fibrosis, the commonest cause of chronic, suppurative lung disease in the UK, affecting 1 in 2000 live births. Many organs are affected, particularly those containing exocrine tissue. Highly viscous secretions cause blockage of the ducts and repeated infections are common. The dental finding shown is due to the incorporation of tetracyline (given to combat recurrent infections) into the forming tooth tissues and retained in the dentine. It is suggested that this photo-oxidises to the red-purple $4\alpha,12\alpha$-anhydro-4-oxo-4-dedimethylaminotetracycline (AODTC).

(b) Present treatment alternatives would appear to be the placement of porcelain veneers at a suitable age or intra-coronal bleaching requiring prior root canal therapy. Some success has been claimed by the manufacturers of external bleaching agents, including carbamide peroxide.

137 (a) The premolar is associated with an evaginated odontome. The odontome has fractured and exposed pulpal tissue. The tooth has subsequently become non-vital with an associated periapical infection.

(b) If the tooth is to be conserved endodontic treatment will be required. The apex of the tooth is open, and prior to obturation of the pulpal chamber a calcific barrier or further apical closure should be encouraged using a non-setting calcium hydroxide paste.

(c) Evaginated odontomes commonly occur bilaterally and within families; therefore, all the other premolar teeth should be carefully examined and wherever possible siblings should also be examined.

138 (a) The probable cause for the symptoms is teething. The bluish swelling is likely to be an eruption haematoma, but less commonly may signify the presence of a true eruption cyst.

(b) Biting on a hard object such as a teething ring or non-sweetened rusk appears to relieve the discomfort of teething. This may be supplemented with use of a suitable analgesic such as elixir of paracetamol (sugar-free) for a few days. Teething solutions and gels for local application are available, but some are sweetened and their prolonged use is potentially cariogenic. Some also contain local anaesthetic agents and carry a further risk of sensitising the child. Eruption haematomas resolve spontaneously with the emergence of the underlying tooth within a few weeks. Eruption cysts also often rupture spontaneously without any need for treatment. Surgical intervention is needed only if the swelling interferes with normal feeding and involves removal of a portion of the cyst wall.

139 (a) A well-circumscribed, flat, circular, brown pigmented area approximately 1.5 mm in diameter on the mucosa of the hard palate, lying 5 mm from the palatal aspect of the left upper primary second molar.

(b) *Local causes*:
> Ephelis (freckle)
> Amalgam tattoo
> Naevus
> Peutz–Jeghers syndrome
> Pigmented neuro-ectodermal tumour of infancy
> Malignant melanoma
> Kaposi's sarcoma

General causes:
> Racial
> Jaundice
> Drugs, e.g. anti-malarial, phenothiazines
> Irritation, e.g. smoking
> Fibrous dysplasia
> Addison's disease
> Albright's syndrome
> Incontinentia pigmentii
> Haemochromatosis
> Von Recklinghausen's disease
> Heavy metal intoxication

(c) This lesion had been noticed before by the patient. It was symptomless and had not changed at all in appearance. It is likely to be an ephelis but could be a pigmented naevus. It was decided to manage this patient on a regular review basis, but excision biopsy has been recommended in cases of pigmented naevi in order to exclude malignancy and because of the premalignant potential of the junctional naevus.

140 (a) Ehlers–Danlos syndrome.
(b) There is an increased incidence of mitral valve prolapse, of dissecting aortic aneurysms and of other arterial rupture. The skin is hyperextensible and is thin and fragile, and there is marked hypermobility of the joints as shown here.
(c) There may be the characteristic ability to touch the nose with the tip of the tongue; this is found is approximately 50% of those with Ehlers–Danlos syndrome but less than 10% of the general population. Various eye problems including myopia, retinal detachment and blue sclerae have been noted. The oral mucosa is fragile and easily bruised, so that suturing is difficult and wound closure may be a problem. Periodontal disease has been reported at an early age. Recurrent sub-luxation of the temporo-mandibular joint occurs. On radiographs there may be evidence of stunted and deformed roots with large pulp stones coronally.

141 (a) Conical, tuberculate, supplemental, odontomes.

(b) There are six erupted incisors, four of which resemble central incisors.

(c) Extraction of the more distal 'central incisor' on each side and alignment of the remaining incisors by means of a fixed appliance.

142 (a) The radiograph shows a root-filled tooth which has a middle third root fracture.

(b) The tooth suffered trauma and became non-vital when it was immature. The root filling was placed after first inducing an apical barrier using calcium hydroxide paste. A further minor trauma has resulted in the root fracture. It is not unusual to find that immature root-filled teeth suffer crown/root fractures after only minor trauma. This is thought to be because these teeth are brittle following root canal therapy and there is little tooth structure due to loss of vitality, and hence lack of dentine deposition at a young age.

(c) The crown and root need to be removed. If the patient is old enough an implant can be considered; otherwise, a denture/composite etch retained bridge will need to be made.

143 (a) These grossly hyperplastic gingivae are likely to be associated with drug therapy. Phenytoin has been known to cause hyperplasia for some time. This is an anticonvulsant drug used for epilepsy. More recently cyclosporin, an immunosuppressive agent, has been found to be associated with hyperplasia. This has particular use in the field of organ and tissue transplantation for prevention of graft rejection following bone marrow, kidney, liver, pancreas, heart and heart lung transplantation, and for prophylaxis of graft versus host disease. It has other major side-effects including hypertrichosis which can also be seen in this patient. Two other drugs associated with gingival swelling are nifedipine, an antihypertensive drug, and diltiazem, an antianginal drug. Both of these are calcium channel blockers, interfering with the inward displacement of calcium ions through the slow channels of active cell membranes. The patient illustrated has received a renal transplant and was being treated with both cyclosporin to prevent rejection and nifedipine to control his blood pressure.

(b) The degree of hyperplasia may have some relationship to the dosage and length of time of administration of cyclosporin—research evidence is somewhat conflicting. At present, however, it is likely that patients who have had kidney transplants will always be on a maintenance dose. Children who have undergone liver transplantation have their dosage gradually reduced and then withdrawn. The cyclosporin dosage for this particular patient could not be reduced. He was, therefore, treated by (i) intensive oral hygiene instruction; (ii) sub-gingival irrigation with chlorhexidine solution; (iii) surgical reduction of hyperplastic tissue; and (iv) reinforcement of oral hygiene measures.

144 (a) Serial extraction is the planned extraction of certain primary teeth followed by the removal of first premolars, to encourage spontaneous correction of incisor crowding.

(b) (i) All primary canines are extracted at the time that the upper lateral incisors begin to erupt, usually at around 8 years of age. (ii) All first primary molars are extracted one year later. (iii) The first premolars are extracted as the permanent canine begins to erupt.

(c) (i) To provide space for spontaneous decrowding of incisors. (ii) To encourage the first premolars to erupt before the canines. (iii) To provide space in the arch into which the canines can erupt.

(d) (i) The child must undergo repeated extraction of teeth. (ii) Uncontrolled space loss may mean that even following the extractions, insufficient space remains to permit proper canine alignment.

145 (a) Chlorhexidine as a 0.2% mouthrinse.

(b) It is a cationic compound that binds to the hydroxyapatite of tooth enamel, pellicle, plaque bacteria, extra-cellular polysaccharides of plaque and to oral mucosa. The chlorhexidine absorbed to the hydroxyapatite is believed to inhibit bacterial colonisation. After binding, the agent is slowly released in active form over a 12–24 hour period.

(c) This patient has composite restorations in both upper central incisors which have become stained, particularly at the margins. These will need to be replaced. A professional prophylaxis will also be required. Advice can then be given to use a conventional toothpaste and remove all plaque *before* using the chlorhexidine mouthrinse in future. This will minimise stain formation but may not entirely prevent it.

146 (a) Cleidocranial dysplasia.

(b) Autosomal dominant, but occasionally it can arise spontaneously.

(c) Aplasia or hypoplasia of clavicles, abnormally wide cranium, delayed ossification of fontanelles, excessive number of wormian bones, hypoplastic pelvis.

(d) Prolonged or permanent delay of eruption of many teeth, dentigerous cysts are frequently found. Many supernumerary teeth may be found, especially in the anterior mandible; these usually remain buried.

147 (a) In addition to the usual history and examination, an effort must be made to account for the missing tooth fragments. The possibility that the fragments are in the lungs must not be overlooked. Therefore, the child and the accompanying adult must be asked if there has been loss of consciousness, if the fragments could have been inhaled or if there is a persistent cough.

(b) Periapical radiographs of the incisors should be taken to check for pathology, root fractures and stage of root development. The lower lip, which is obviously traumatised, must be radiographed to look for the missing fragments. If there is suspicion that a tooth fragment has been inhaled the child should be referred to hospital for a chest radiograph.

(c) A soft-tissue radiograph of the lower lip shows the presence of tooth fragments which should be removed under local anaesthesia. The fractured incisors must be treated by covering the exposed dentine with a calcium hydroxide liner followed by an acid-etch composite restoration. An alternative treatment would be to bond the fragment back onto the tooth using a dentine bonding agent.

148 Routine dental treatment may involve one or all of these different techniques, depending on the child's maturity and ability to co-operate. (a) Tell-show-do, in which each part of treatment is explained and demonstrated before proceeding, is often used routinely and is of value once a child is sufficiently mature to understand and co-operate with instructions. Even in this case, it is important that the method be used gently and slowly with explanations that are suitable for the child's level of understanding.

(b) In the absence of contra-indications local anaesthesia should be used routinely for restorative treatment, once the child is able to understand and tolerate the loss of sensation involved. Painless administration (through such measures as the use of topical anaesthetic, a warmed cartridge and a skilful and gentle technique) is essential if local anaesthesia is to be well accepted by the young child. A co-operative and relaxed young child may accept both restorative care and extractions of teeth with local anaesthetic alone; but in other cases, particularly where multiple extractions are indicated, inhalational sedation or general anaesthesia may be required.

(c) Inhalational sedation may not be suitable for the very young child who is unable to understand the change in sensation or who cannot co-operate sufficiently to use the nasal mask. However, for some more mature children, inhalational sedation may be of great value in overcoming anxiety and in completing more complex and radical treatments.

(d) General anaesthesia, under 'day bed' facilities or with hospital admission, may be the preferred option for the child who is too young to be able to co-operate with other techniques. It may also be especially suitable for the child needing large amounts of treatment including both restorations and multiple extractions.

149 (a) Fusion of the upper primary central and lateral incisor teeth.

(b) Presence of the permanent central incisor and absence of the permanent lateral incisor.

(c) Extraction of the fused primary teeth as soon as possible. It would have been advisable for these teeth to have been extracted at the time that the upper right permanent central incisor was erupting. Assessment of the dentition will be necessary as the other permanent teeth erupt, in order to decide whether to close the space or replace the missing incisor tooth.

150 (a) The child has been persistently scratching at the gingiva on the lower right central incisor.

(b) Gingivitis artefacta.

(c) Treat the local irritation; some sub-gingival calculus was present and this should be removed and root planing carried out followed by intensive oral hygiene instruction. Both the child and the parents were counselled. If the habit persists this may be an indication of an underlying psychiatric disorder and psychiatric help may be required in severe cases.

151 (a) There has been marked replacement resorption of the previously root-filled right upper central incisor. There is root-canal obliteration in the right lateral and left central incisors.

(b) The most likely scenario is that the upper anterior teeth were traumatised and the right central incisor was avulsed and replanted. The tooth was subsequently root-filled but is undergoing slow replacement resorption.

(c) It is unlikely that this tooth is mobile because this type of resorption involves replacement of the resorbed root by bone with the probability of ankylosis and reduced mobility.

(d) No treatment is indicated. The likely outcome is that the resorbed tooth will eventually exhibit sudden mobility following minor trauma which destroys the attachment of the remaining root to the bone. At that stage its extraction and replacement, initially by a denture, must be accepted.

152 (i) Detailed medical history to eliminate systemic factors. (ii) Full clinical examination including pocket depth measurement. (iii) Radiographic assessment: an orthopantomogram with periapical radiographs of upper and lower incisors. This would show bone levels and any evidence of other boney pathology. (iv) Haematological screening: assess for presence of anaemia, leukaemia, neutropenia, etc. (v) Biopsy: this may not be required for this patient but would depend on the results from the other investigations.

153 (a) Fibrous tissue with a dense infiltrate of inflammatory cells. Numerous eosinophils are present but the majority of the inflammatory cells are histiocytes.
(b) Histiocytosis X. This is an uncommon group of diseases characterised by the infiltration or proliferation of histiocytes in various body tissues. It has been sub-divided into three groups: a localised form known as eosinophilic granuloma; a chronic disseminated type known as Hand–Schüller–Christian disease; and an acute form which occurs in early infancy and is referred to as Letterer–Siwe disease. Initial signs and symptoms which may lead to diagnosis are frequently noted in the oral cavity. The pre-pubertal periodontitis shown in this patient is often associated with systemic conditions such as diabetes, hyper-parathyroidism, adrenocortical insufficiency, scleroderma, or as in this case, with histiocytosis X.

154 (a) Amelogenesis imperfecta, hypoplastic type.
(b) It is an inherited condition; this young girl shows an autosomal dominant mode of inheritance of this hypoplastic type. The main classification is into hypoplastic, hypocalcified and hypomaturation forms, with subclassification based on the mode of inheritance.
(c) She complains of the appearance but also of sensitivity to hot and cold substances.

155 In Westernised societies, non-milk extrinsic sugars are believed to represent the most important dietary factor in caries. Sucrose is considered the most important of these, but glucose, fructose and maltose are thought to be only marginally less cariogenic. Staple starchy foods, intrinsic sugars (for example those contained within the cell structure of whole fruits and milk sugars) are thought to be negligible causes of dental caries. Non-sugar bulk and intense sweeteners are non-cariogenic or virtually so.

156 (a) Diet has a very minor role in the aetiology, prevention and treatment of periodontal disease. Many nutrients have been shown to adversely affect periodontal tissues in animal experiments but these effects have not been observed in man.
(b) Only vitamin C deficiency (scurvy) clearly involves the gingival tissues. Some recent evidence indicates that folate applied locally to the gingivae may reduce gingivitis in subjects susceptible to folate deficiency in 'end-tissues' such as gingivae.

157 (a) The crowns of the right upper primary central and lateral incisors have been displaced palatally. The radiograph shows that there are no root fractures evident. The anterior open bite means that there is no interference with occlusion.
(b) The child is 4 years old.
(c) No active treatment is needed. The parent should be instructed to give the child a soft diet with plenty of fluids and to keep the traumatised teeth clean using chlorhexidine mouthwash on a swab twice daily. The periodontal ligament and gingivae around the central and lateral incisors will heal in 1–2 weeks. The displaced teeth will usually regain their original position due to tongue and lip forces.
(d) There is always the possibility that trauma to a primary tooth may damage the permanent successor. However, it is unlikely in this instance because the roots for the right upper central and lateral incisors have been displaced buccally, away from the permanent tooth germs. This is in contrast to the situation where the crowns are displaced buccally and the roots, therefore, rotate palatally and come into direct contact with the permanent teeth, and when intrusion of the primary incisors occurs.

158 (a) Investigate the fluoride intake during the period of tooth development and check the medical history for systemic disturbances such as exanthematous fevers.
(b) Treatment with a controlled acid-pumice enamel abrasion technique (micro-abrasion) may prove effective for this patient. A localised thin layer of composite may be required.

159 (a) There are two inverted supernumerary teeth of the conical or mesiodens form. There appears to be insufficient space for the eruption of the permanent lateral incisors.
(b) None at present. Surgical removal of the supernumerary teeth at this stage may cause damage to the blood supply of the developing permanent incisor teeth. There should be regular radiographic reviews and surgery should be undertaken if pathological changes develop.

160 (a) A talon cusp—a morphologically well-delineated cusp that projects from the lingual surface of a primary or permanent anterior tooth and extends at least half the distance from the cemento–enamel junction to the incisal edge.
(b) Children who have talon cusps affecting primary incisors commonly have other dental anomalies present. However, it is rare for the permanent successor to be affected in a similar manner. Primary incisors with a talon cusp usually exfoliate uneventfully; a process of selective grinding can be undertaken if the cusp is causing occlusal interference.

161 (a) Haematological—routine screen including iron, folate and vitamin B12 levels; gastro-intestinal—may include jejunal biopsy; oral biopsy—if any mucosal lesions, or of lips.
(b) Crohn's disease. This is a granulomatous disorder of unknown origin, but often with a family history as with this boy. It mainly affects the ileum but can affect any part of the gastro-intestinal tract. Oral features include ulceration, particularly in the buccal sulcus where this may appear with thickening and folding of the mucosa to form a characteristic 'cobblestone' appearance. The lips may swell chronically with splitting and angular cheilitis.
(c) Investigations are required, particularly to exclude sarcoidosis. Topical cortico-steroids may control the lesions but systemic corticosteroids, azathioprine or salazopyrine may be required. Some patients with these oral lesions have been found to be allergic to various food stuffs and colouring agents, and exclusion diets have been used with some success.

162 (a) There is a supernumerary tooth which closely resembles the teeth of the group to which it belongs. In the primary dentition supernumeraries are usually supplemental in form, although they are more common adjacent to the maxillary lateral incisors rather than the central incisors, as in this patient.
(b) The prevalence is 0.2–0.8% in primary dentition.
(c) Ninety per cent of all supernumerary teeth occur in the maxilla.
(d) Autosomal dominant, with incomplete penetrance. Some generations may be unaffected.

163 (a) The vast majority of young children do have snacks and/or drinks between their main meal times and most have these at least 3–4 times a day.
(b) The most popular snacks probably include sweet biscuits, fresh fruit and crisps; diluted fruit squash, carbonated drinks and milk are the most popular drinks. Sweet

biscuits, diluted fruit squash and carbonated drinks are potentially cariogenic, although parents may see them as less harmful than confectionery which is eaten as a snack less often by most children.

(c) Raw fresh fruit and milk are not believed to be important in the development of caries, and may be suitable to recommend as alternative items for eating and drinking between meals. Other suitable substitute foods include savoury sandwiches and crispbreads, pitta bread, natural yoghurt with fresh fruit, cereal (without sugar) with milk, cottage cheese and plain popcorn. Milk or water form the best drinks for use between mealtimes. Fruit juices may have a high natural sugar content and thus be cariogenic. They may also pose an additional risk in terms of enamel erosion because of their high acidity.

164 (a)   Fibro-epithelial polyp
          Pyogenic granuloma
          Fibroma
          Papilloma
          Haematoma from trauma
          Vesiculobullous lesions
          Giant cell lesion
          Oral Crohn's disease

(b) The appearance is suggestive of repeated trauma from biting the buccal mucosa, producing a fibro-epithelial polyp.

(c) An excision biopsy. This confirmed the provisional diagnosis of a fibro-epithelial polyp, and showed a well-keratinised stratified squamous epithelium overlying thick collagenous bundles in the connective tissue, with an inflammatory component.

165 (a) Dilaceration of upper incisor at crown/root junction.

(b) Severe injury to primary incisors between 2 and 5 years of age, by either an intrusive luxation or exarticulation.

(c) (i) Surgical removal and space management. (ii) Exposure and packing: following eruption attempt orthodontic alignment. (iii) Exposure and bonding of chain to undertake orthodontic alignment.

166 (a) Internal or intradental resorption. The lesion has become so extensive that the coronal enamel has been perforated.

(b) In the first instance it may be worthwhile to attempt to arrest the resorptive process by carrying out a partial coronal pulpotomy since the child is very young to lose a first permanent molar. If this treatment is unsuccessful, so that resorption continues or the pulp becomes infected, the tooth must be extracted. In this situation the need to balance the extraction by removing the contralateral tooth should be considered.

167 No. There is evidence that it affects food choice, but not that it adversely affects nutritional intake or health. The quality of complete dentures also affects food choice so that people with no dentures or poorly fitting dentures avoid meat. Fixed prostheses improve biting force and food choice, but there is no evidence that they improve nutrition or health.

168 (a) Odontodysplasia or 'ghost tooth'.

(b) (i) Abnormal vascular supply. (ii) Viral infection. (iii) Genetic causes.

169 (a) Neonatal teeth. A rare occurrence in which teeth are present at birth (natal) or soon after birth (neonatal). Such teeth have been described at 26 weeks' gestation.
(b) Lower incisors of the normal primary dentition.
(c) Ulceration of the infant's tongue, or of the mother's breast if the infant is suckling.
(d) Extractions are best restricted to those teeth that are supernumeraries, or are very loose and in danger of being inhaled.

170 (a) The mandibular permanent left lateral incisor has erupted in an ectopic position, between the primary canine and second primary molar.
(b) Extraction, as part of an orthodontic treatment plan, is the only reasonable treatment. The permanent canine will be positioned mesially to the ectopic lateral incisor so that alignment of the latter cannot be achieved.

171 (a) Pemphigus vulgaris. The anterior aspect of the left maxillary lesion still contains an intra-epithelial vesicle. There is separation of epithelial cells due to loss of inter-epithelial attachment, and this results in ulceration.
(b) It is caused by circulating auto-antibodies against epithelial intercellular substance. Immunoglobulin and complement are localised along intercellular boundaries.
(c) Acantholytic cells in smears from vesicle fluid. Confirmed by biopsy and immunofluoresence microscopy.
(d) Systemic corticosteriods or immunosuppressives are essential and usually life-saving.

172 (a) Loss of bone support.
(b) Maintenance of good oral hygiene; curretage of the defect; irrigation of the pocket with saline; chlorhexidine mouthwash for rinsing.

173 (a) Sugars are introduced into the diet at any early age in both foods and drinks. Sugars, in the form of sucrose, glucose or honey, are sometimes added to milk feeds, a practice that is especially prevalent amongst Asian families as a means of encouraging milk consumption. Sugars are also sometimes given in the form of sweetened water to prevent or treat constipation. Manufactured drinks may not have sugar added as such, but the concentrated fruit juices which form part or whole of the ingredients often have a high natural sugar content. Amongst foods, sugars are added to a proportion of manufactured weaning foods, especially rusks and non-fruit dessert items. Some mothers also introduce sweet biscuits and confectionery to their child's diet at an early age.
(b) The significance of sugars present in the diet at weaning lies partly in their direct effect on caries affecting erupted teeth. However, frequent use of sweet items also encourages a liking for, and a habit of eating, sweet foods and drinks. That this does occur is shown in a study in which a correlation was demonstrated between the use of sweetened comforters in infancy and the consumption of sugar-containing snacks in later life.

174 (a) Prolonged use of a dummy or feeding bottle, or persistent thumb or finger sucking.
(b) Cessation of the dummy habit before the loss of the lower primary incisors. The permanent incisor teeth should then erupt into an acceptable occlusion.

175 (a) There appears to be a conical supernumerary tooth erupting buccally to the upper right permanent central incisor tooth.
(b) Radiographs of (i) periapical parallax views of the upper central incisors; (ii) an

orthopantomogram to check whether there are any other dental anomalies or pathology. Careful clinical investigations of the relationship of the supernumerary tooth to the central incisor.
(c) Extraction of the supernumerary tooth.
(d) This supernumerary element was completely fused to the buccal aspect of the root of the central incisor. It required a surgical approach to dissect the conical supernumerary element from the permanent incisor.

176 (a) The tooth has been restored with a crown of radio-opaque material. The root shows external inflammatory resorption along the lateral aspects. The apical development of the tooth is complete and there appears to be a small area of periapical radiolucency.
(b) After measuring, cleaning and shaping the canal to arrest root resorption, calcium hydroxide should be applied. On stabilisation of the situation, a root filling should be placed with gutta-percha and sealer. The crown should be restored following assessment of the extent of tissue loss.

177 (a) Pebbly or cobblestone proliferation. This is a thickening and folding of the mucosa with purple granulomatous enlargement appearing on the gingiva.
(b) Crohn's disease.
(c) Orofacial granulomatosis.
(d) Histologically, the epithelium is intact but thickened, with epithelioid cells and giant cells surrounded by a lymphocytic infiltration. This appearance is characteristic of chronic granulomatous disease.

178 (a) Patients with cystic fibrosis (CF) usually have a restricted intake of dietary fat. To compensate for loss of energy from fat, they are encouraged to eat high carbohydrate diets.
(b) Protein intake may be restricted in patients with phenylketonuria (PKU) and these patients may also be encouraged to consume high carbohydrate diets.
(c) Consumption of sugar by diabetics is no longer severely restricted, but they are encouraged to eat starch rather than sugars and to eat regularly. Dentists should discuss dietary advice with the physicians of diabetics concerned and not alter diets of those patients without full agreement. The high carbohydrate diets of patients with CF and PKU will mean that non-dietary caries-preventive measures become very important.

179 (a) Ankylosis or infra-occlusion.
(b) Replacement resorption of the root.
(c) Extraction becomes more difficult. The adjacent teeth may tilt mesially with the loss of contact points and space. The opposing tooth may over-erupt. The gingival margin may be at a much higher level than the adjacent tooth, so that prosthetic replacement with a bridge may be very difficult and a denture or implant may be necessary.

180 This child had bitten his tongue severely and there was some tissue loss and ulceration present. He did not appear to be suffering any discomfort. He has the rare syndrome of congenital indifference (insensitivity) to pain. Absence of appropriate responses to painful stimuli is found as an isolated abnormality in an otherwise healthy child. However, there are significant problems with this condition as failure to appreciate pain leads to repeated skin trauma and burns, as well as to the infant biting himself as shown here. In some patients the condition is distinguishable from the recessively inherited congenital sensory neuropathy by the universal absence of pain sensation but the preservation of touch, position, vibration and temperature senses.

181 (a) Infra-occlusion of the second primary molar.
(b) Radiographs to ascertain the presence and position of the second pre-molar and the rest of the permanent dentition.
(c) If the second pre-molar is present, the second primary molar should be extracted if it is *not* exfoliated at the time of eruption of the contralateral second pre-molar. Many infra-occluded teeth are shed normally. If there is absence of the second pre-molar, an orthodontic assessment should be made to decide whether or not it is desirable to retain the space for replacement of the missing tooth, or whether the space should be closed orthodontically. Any tooth that shows evidence of infra-occlusion requires regular monitoring.

182 Only (d) implies that a product has been specifically tested for cariogenicity and found to have little or no effect on plaque pH levels. (c) may also show low cariogenicity, although plaque pH studies have suggested some starch products to be potentially cariogenic. At present, in the case of both (a) and (b), products may still contain relatively high levels of sugar and still be potentially cariogenic.

183 (a) An epulis, probably fibrous in origin. The term 'epulis' is now applied to any lump arising from gingival tissue. The fibrous epulis resembles a fibro-epithelial polyp, but usually also has an inflammatory component.
(b) In view of the age of the child this lesion should be kept under review, and if no change is observed an excision biopsy under local anaesthesia should be carried out when the primary molar tooth is due to be exfoliated. Fibrous epulides should be removed down to the periosteum and curetted thoroughly.

184 (a) Cherubism (familial fibrous dysplasia).
(b) Autosomal dominant.
(c) Loose vascular connective tissue with giant cells.
(d) Mandibular swelling appears at about 2–4 years of age, proceeding slowly until becoming relatively static at around 8–10 years. The deformity never disappears but usually arrests or regresses after puberty.
(e) (i) Clinical features; (ii) radiological appearances; (iii) histopathology; (iv) behaviour of lesion.

185 (a) Supernumerary teeth
Dentigerous cyst associated with unerupted permanent tooth
Dilaceration of unerupted permanent tooth root
Abnormal collection of unerupted dental tissue—odontome
Local bone or soft tissue pathology
Congenital absence of permanent incisor (very rare)
(b) 6–9 months.

186 (a) (i) How, when and where did the accident happen? (ii) General medical history. This is a rather bizarre type of injury with the left upper primary central and lateral incisors completely displaced from their sockets in a buccal direction and the right incisors subluxed and displaced palatally. However, the explanation given by the parent was quite consistent with the injuries seen. If the explanation is inconsistent, and particularly if there is delay in reporting the injury, then the possibility of non-accidental injury should always be considered.
(b) These teeth will require extraction under general anaesthetic.

187 (a) Yes. Liquid medicines which contain sugar can be an aetiological factor in dental caries.
(b) Some syrup-based medicines contain up to 60% sucrose, glucose and fructose.
(c) Dental caries caused by liquid medicines can be prevented if sugar-free medicines are prescribed by doctors and if the parents buy the sugar-free varieties from their pharmacist.
(d) The commonly used alternative sweeteners in sugar-free medicines are hydrogenated glucose syrup, sorbitol and saccharin.

188 Children who are teething often find that biting on hard objects (for example teething rings) gives relief. Teething gels can be recommended as they give local pain relief. All teething gels should now be sugar-free. A sugar-free paracetamol elixir can also be recommended.

189 (a) An upper right central incisor with a restoration, possibly of amalgam in a probable access cavity; a sclerosed but fine root canal; periapical root resorption; loss of lamina dura around root and replacement resorption distally.
(b) A luxation injury.
(c) Endodontic therapy with calcium hydroxide to attempt to arrest the resorption process.

190 (a) Talon cusp.
(b) Ninety per cent in the maxillary and 90% in the anterior permanent teeth.
(c) Unknown, but have been known to occur with other dental anomalies such as odontomes and impacted maxillary canines.
(d) (i) They may be seen radiographically prior to eruption and mistaken for a supernumerary tooth. (ii) They may interfere with occlusion by forming a premature contact, which may lead to damage and pain in the periodontal ligament, or even displacement of the tooth. (iii) The cusp or opposing tooth may undergo attrition. (iv) Interference with tongue space: speech may be affected, the tongue may be irritated. (v) Aesthetic problems. (vi) Plaque retention and increased risk of dental caries.

191 (a) Cyclosporin, nifedipine.
(b) Phenytoin.
(c) The exact mechanism of drug interaction is unknown. There is proliferation of subgingival collagen, mainly of the interdental papillae which become grossly swollen, pale and firm with enhanced orange-peel stippling. Hyperplasia is more pronounced when oral hygiene is poor.

192 (a) A partial pulpotomy was carried out following a coronal fracture which resulted in a small pulpal exposure. The radiopaque calcium hydroxide paste can be seen at the pulpotomy site.

(b) Yes. There has been continued root maturation and apical closure. In addition, a calcific barrier is visible at the pulpotomy site.

(c) The tooth will usually respond to vitality tests because the coronal pulp remains, unlike a cervical pulpotomy where the coronal pulp is removed. The presence of vital pulp in the coronal pulp chamber means that dentine will continue to be laid down. This is in contrast to a cervical pulpotomy which leaves a brittle crown which is easily fractured if further trauma occurs.

(d) The reported success rate for partial pulpotomy is 96%.

193 All non-sugar sweeteners have been considered by the Committee on Toxicology (COT) of foods in the Department of Health and found to be safe for the inclusion in foods. However, some non-sugar sweeteners have disadvantages including: (i) cost—most are more expensive than sugars, although saccharine is much cheaper than sugar for similar levels of sweetness; (ii) taste—saccharine has a bitter taste to most people; (iii) intestinal upset—the polyols (sorbitol, mannitol, lactitol and xylitol) are poorly absorbed and tend to cause osmotic diarrhoea. This can be a problem, especially in children. High consumption levels should be avoided, although subjects in the Turku studies ate over 100 g/day without adverse symptoms; (iv) phenylketonuria (PKU)—aspartame contains phenylalanine, intake of which should be restricted by people with PKU; (v) lack of fermentability—this very property ensures they are 'safe for teeth' but can cause bakers a problem.

194 (a) A salivary calculus.

(b) Although salivary calculus formation is relatively common in adults, it is rare in childhood. Haematological and biochemical screening for alkaline phosphatase levels should, therefore, be carried out.

(c) It may be possible to remove the calculus by bimanual palpation to 'milk' the stone from the salivary duct. If this is unsuccessful, then surgical removal may be necessary.

195 (a) The orthodontic wire has been attached to the teeth using an acid-etch composite technique. This has been used to give rigidity of the root-fractured tooth in order to facilitate hard tissue union between the apical and coronal tooth portions. If movement of the right central incisor occurs this would favour soft tissue/fibrous union.

(b) Three months.

(c) Conscientious use of the chlorhexidine mouthwash, which was prescribed to aid plaque control around the splint.

196 (a) Left and right rotated lateral oblique radiographs (bimolars).

(b) Between 6.5 and 7 years.

(c) Impaction of maxillary first permanent molars and extensive root resorption of second primary molars.

(d) Crowding in the maxilla.

(e) There is already very extensive root resorption on the second primary molars so they will either exfoliate shortly or will require to be extracted to allow the first permanent molars to erupt. Orthodontic treatment will be required subsequently to de-crowd the maxilla.

197 (a) There is extensive erosion of the palatal dental hard tissues with areas of exposed sensitive dentine.

(b) The likely aetiological factor is gastro-oesophageal reflux. This has been found to be common in people with a mental handicap and several possible contributory factors have been identified. These are extension spasms, inco-ordination of deglutition, kyphosis, scoliosis and prolonged recumbency; all of these factors may be present in people with cerebral palsy.

(c) Dental care should be directed towards preventing further erosion and eliminating pain. Study casts are useful for accurate monitoring of on-going tooth tissue loss. Liaison with the general medical practitioner may enable the reflux oesophagitis to be controlled by various preparations, including an alginate which forms a foaming agent on the gastric contents, metoclopramide hydrochloride to improve oesophageal mobility and sphincter function, or H2 antagonists such as cimetidine. A vacuum-formed splint filled with magnesium hydroxide or sodium bicarbonate may be of value if worn during danger periods to help neutralise the acidic effects of the reflux activity. Exposed dentine should be covered if possible by one of the glass ionomer cements or dentine bonding agents. A concentrated fluoride varnish such as Duraphat is also useful to minimise sensitivity.

198 Sugarless gums improve dental health, but sugar-containing gums do not. Clinical trials have recorded no improvement in gingival health in children who chewed gum. Children who chewed sugared gum regularly developed more dental caries than those who did not chew gum. Children and adults who chewed sugarless gum developed less dental caries than those who either chewed no gum or who chewed sugared gum.

199 (a) Lichen planus
Leukoplakia
—idiopathic
—candidal
—syphilitic
Benign migratory glossitis

(b) History, clinical features, presence of skin lesions, biopsy. The dorsum of the tongue is a characteristic site for lichen planus, although a biopsy may show classical histopathological features; often the histological and immunological findings are reported as 'consistent with lichen planus'.

(c) Any drugs implicated in the aetiology of lichen planus should be changed. Topical corticosteriods are often effective in the control of lesions; rarely, systemic corticosteroids may be required.

200 (a) (i) Amelogenesis imperfecta: hypoplastic type. (ii) Gross caries in maxillary first permanent molars. (iii) Unerupted upper canines with no space for them in the dental arch. (iv) Right upper lateral incisor palatally displaced—'inside the bite'. (v) Gingival inflammation, particularly in lower incisor region, associated with inadequate oral hygiene.

(b) Family history investigation; this might identify the mode of inheritance of the amelogenesis imperfecta. Radiographs are required to identify the position and presence of the unerupted canine and molar teeth. An orthopantomogram and parallax views to localise the canine would be helpful.

(c) The patient probably is not concerned about his appearance. He has never attended a dentist before so his motivation for extensive dental treatment is doubtful. Therefore, a suggested treatment plan would include (i) extraction of upper first permanent molars; (ii) identification of position of upper canines. These were ectopically placed and lying in the palate. It was decided to leave them *in situ* and monitor them radiographically; (iii) desensitisation; application of fluoride varnish and use of fluoride-containing desensitising toothpaste; (iv) oral hygiene instruction and dietary advice; (v) reassessment —orthodontic treatment to correct the position of the right upper lateral incisor could be considered but this would depend on motivation and co-operation of the patient.

201 (a) Osteogenesis imperfecta.
(b) Affected individuals have repeated bony fractures following minimal trauma, sometimes from birth, with progressive deafness and joint laxity. Skull radiographs usually show evidence of wormian bones.
c) This condition may be associated with dentinogenesis imperfecta (same patient as in *Figure 31*).

202 Many different types of microorganism have been shown to be capable of producing caries in experimental animals. The two bacterial species that have most commonly been associated with caries in children are *Lactobacilli* and *Streptococcus mutans*. *Lactobacilli* are now often thought to be opportunists, with more attention being focused on *S. mutans*. However, even in this case, evidence is not clearcut. There have been suggestions that species may be strongly affected by the presence of others, so that caries may represent the outcome of a 'micro-community' rather than the effects of a single species.

203 (a) Bohn's nodules.
(b) Along the midpalatine raphe. These are known as 'Epstein's pearls'. They are reported to be present in about 60–80% of neonates.
(c) Bohn's nodules are found on the maxillary and mandibular ridges and are cysts derived from the dental lamina. Epstein's pearls, although they appear to be similar, arise from embryologically trapped epithelium and are, therefore, histologically different.
(d) The mother should be reassured; active treatment is unnecessary as they are shed spontaneously within a few weeks.

204 (a) Sturge–Weber syndrome (encephalo-trigeminal angiomatosis).
(b) The halitosis may be related to poor oral hygiene exacerbated by difficulties in cleaning the affected haemangiomatous area. Acute ulcerative gingivitis causes a particularly marked breath odour. Intensive oral hygiene instruction with scaling and polishing should be carried out and the use of a chlorhexidine mouthwash and spray should be suggested.
(c) Uncontrollable haemorrhage from the haemangioma may be a problem. The Sturge–Weber syndrome is often associated with epilepsy and hemiparesis on the side opposite the lesion. Angioma in the choroid may lead to glaucoma in childhood.

205 (a) This is most likely to be a pyogenic granuloma, an excessive granulation-tissue response to trauma or infection. Initial growth is quite rapid and they are red, elevated and easily traumatised. Histological examination shows granulation tissue with marked endothelial proliferation forming vascular channels and a dense polymorphonuclear leucocyte infiltrate.

(b) Treatment consists of excision with scalpel or electocautery. However, recurrence is common unless the causative irritant, usually calculus or foreign material, is removed.

206 As in young children, prevention of caries in adolescents may be achieved partly through appropriate use of fluorides and through dietary modification. (a) Fluoride supplements are thought to be of reduced value in this age group, although they may still be of some benefit in areas where water levels are less than optimal and where caries risk is very high. (b) Fluoride mouthrinses may be thought to be an appropriate measure that may provide some extra benefit even with the use of fluoride toothpaste. Mouthrinses may be particularly valuable in children undergoing orthodontic treatment. (c) Achieving dietary modification requires a very different approach in adolescents. Good communication skills and an understanding approach are needed. (d) Oral hygiene instructions are of great value in preventing gingivitis, but they do not represent a means of preventing caries in adolescents. Toothbrushing is a good means of applying fluoride toothpaste but, despite public belief, the effect of brushing alone on caries is probably very limited. (e) Fissure sealing is effective in preventing occlusal caries. Susceptible teeth need to be sealed as soon as possible after eruption before caries can occur. In the young adolescent at risk of developing caries, second permanent molars may well stand to benefit particularly from sealing. First permanent molars that have remained caries-free may profit less, although if one has become carious, sealing may be indicated for the remaining three. Premolar fissures are less susceptible to caries, although sealing may be of benefit to those who are particularly at risk from the consequences of dental disease.

207 (a) These are periapical radiographs showing the presence of:

$$\underline{6\ 4\ 3\ 2\ 1}\ |\ \underline{1\ 2\ 3\ 4\ 6}$$

There is generalised evidence of short root formation, although the first permanent molars and incisors are not as extensively affected as the premolars and canines. This is suggestive of a chronological effect.

(b) (i) Radiotherapy given for a solid tumour at 8–9 years of age. (ii) Chemotherapy given for leukaemia or a solid tumour at the same age. It has now been reported that chemotherapy may have a number of dental effects. Several workers have shown an increased prevalence of enamel hypoplasia and hypodontia as well as altered root development. Radiographic studies demonstrate marked shortening of premolar roots in particular, with thinning of the roots and enlargement of the pulp chambers. (iii) Trauma, although it is theoretically possible that direct trauma to teeth can induce root resorption, this usually occurs following pulp necrosis. There is no evidence from these radiographs that this has occurred. It would also seem to be highly unlikely that trauma could affect so many teeth. (iv) Orthodontic treatment. Root resorption can and does occur during active tooth movement. Excessive pressures or 'jiggling' movements can produce marked tooth resorption, usually in the incisor region. (v) Iatrogenic.

208 (a) This is a fibro-epithelial polyp, and is a result of trauma producing a more vigorous localised tissue overgrowth than is usual in the normal healing process. These fibrous lumps are much more common than truly neoplastic fibromas.

(b) The polyp should be excised with its entire base for histological examination, which will usually show a well-keratinised stratified squamous epithelium, as in this case, overlying a connective tissue with criss-crossing thick collagenous bundles. Inflammatory signs are minimal and there is no capsule.

209 (a) (i) Hemihyperplasia (hemihypertrophy). The aetiology and pathogenesis are poorly understood, but most cases are sporadic. Suggestions have been made that there may be anatomic and functional vascular or lymphatic abnormalities which lead to the development of hyperplasia. Asymmetry is usually present at birth and becomes accentuated with age, particularly at puberty. This condition should be differentiated from neurofibromatosis and Beckwith–Wiedemann syndrome. (ii) Hemifacial atrophy (Romberg syndrome). Slowly progressive atrophy of the soft tissues of half the face. Usually accompanied by contralateral Jacksonian epilepsy. Nearly all cases are sporadic, but there have been several examples of familial instances in the literature. There have also been reports of this occurring following trauma. This condition should be differentiated from scleroderma and fat necrosis. (iii) Hemifacial microsomia. The clinical picture of this condition consists of unusual facial asymmetry with unilateral ear deformity and hypoplasia, especially of the ramus and condyle of the mandible. As with hemihyperplasia and hemifacial atrophy, it usually occurs sporadically. This condition should be differentiated from mandibulofacial dysostosis and Goldenhar syndrome (see **127**).
(b) Obviously, full preventive advice and care are important whatever the diagnosis. In hemihyperplasia, there may be dental anomalies such as megadontia on the affected side. Malocclusion will occur in all conditions and may be untreatable by conventional orthodontics. Various neoplasms, most commonly Wilms' tumour, have been reported in association with hemihyperplasia. In early cases of hemifacial atrophy the temporal and buccinator muscles are affected. This extends to involve the brow, angle of the mouth and neck. Atrophy of half of the upper lip and tongue are characteristic. The teeth on the affected side may be delayed in eruption or have short roots. In hemifacial microsomia there may be hearing impairment.

210 (a) Shortly after the eruption of the upper permanent central incisors, at about the age of 8–8½ years.
(b) Establish drainage through the palatal aspects of the upper left central and lateral incisors. Root-fill these teeth and then enucleate the dental cyst in relation to them. Monitor the vitality of the upper left canine tooth.
(c) If the patient had been seen at regular intervals following the trauma, and regular radiographic examination and vitality tests had been undertaken, the loss of vitality of the left upper incisors would have been detected and they could have been treated endodontically before cyst formation occurred.

211 (a) Major ulceration.
(b) Most of the ulceration occurs in the first 14 weeks following the start of treatment. It appears mainly on the inner margins of the lips, on the cheeks, and on the sides and tip of the tongue. More ulceration is apparent when the neutrophil count is low.
(c) Oral hygiene must be of a high standard and be carefully maintained. Chlorhexidine (0.2%) mouthwashes and sprays should be used. Methotrexate is the chemotherapeutic agent that causes most ulceration but this may be helped by concomitant intravenous administration of folinic acid ('leucovorin rescue'). Amphotericin should be prescribed to prevent candidal infections. The pain from the ulceration can be helped by using benzydamine mouthwash or spray, or using a lignocaine ointment or lozenges.

212 (a) Many drugs currently used in children have not been studied adequately or at all in paediatric patients. All children, particularly in the neonatal period, differ from adults in their response to drugs. Although not ideal, doses are generally based on body weight in kilograms or sometimes in the following age ranges:

first month (neonate)
up to 1 year (infant)
1–5 years
6–12 years.

However, the body surface area method of calculating drug dosages is the most reliable and gives a more consistent dosage. This is calculated from the following formula, with body surface area being taken from standard tables:

$$\text{Dose for patient} = \frac{\text{body surface (in m}^2) \times \text{adult dose}}{1.8}$$

(b) If the patient is not allergic to penicillin (and has not received penicillin or derivatives in the last 28 days) give 1.5 g amoxycillin 1 hour before the procedure. If the patient is allergic to penicillin (or has received it in the preceding 28 days) give 300 mg oral clindamycin 1.5 hours before the procedure.

213 (a) Fracture of the middle third of the root of the upper right permanent central incisor tooth.
(b) A splint should be placed on the tooth for 3 months so that no movement can occur and the vitality monitored. Endodontic treatment should be carried out if the tooth becomes non-vital.

214 (a) Rubella infection of his mother during pregnancy.
(b) Gingival hyperplasia as a result of treatment for his epilepsy by phenytoin.
(c) Initial treatment should be aimed at improving oral hygiene measures. His medical practitioner should be approached regarding change of drug. Gingivectomy may be necessary.

INDEX

Numbers refer to Question and Answer numbers.